Seattle !

MAGNIFIQUE

INSIDE & OUT

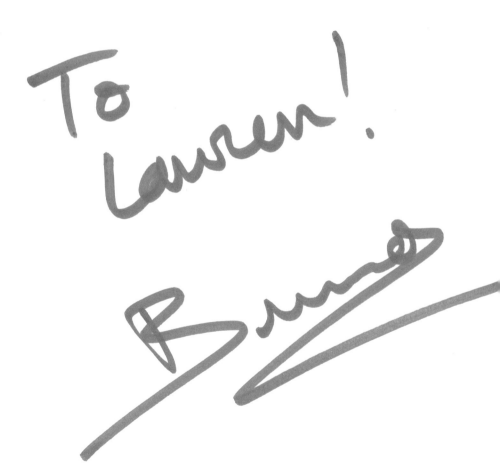

To
Lauren!

Bruno

MAGNIFIQUE

INSIDE & OUT

Find Out How Truly Beautiful You Are

BRUNO GRALPOIS

Waterside Press

Magnifique Inside & Out. Copyright © 2015 by Bruno Gralpois.
All rights reserved. No part of this book may be used or
reproduced in any form or by any electronic or mechanical means,
including photocopying, recording, scanning, information storage and
retrieval systems, without written permission from the publisher, except
in the case of brief quotations embodied in articles and reviews.

Limit of Liability/Disclaimer of Warranty: While the publisher and
author have used their best efforts in preparing this book, they make
no representations or warranties with respect to the accuracy or
completeness of the contents of this book and specifically disclaim any
implied warranties of merchantability or fitness for a particular purpose.
No warranty may be created or extended by sales representatives or written
sales materials. The advice and strategies contained herein may not be suitable
for your situation. You should consult with a professional where appropriate.
Neither the publisher nor author shall be liable for any loss of profit or any other
commercial damages, including but not limited to special, incidental, conse-
quential, or other damages. Readers should be aware that Internet sites offered
as citations and/or sources for further information may have changed or disap-
peared between the time this was written and when it is read.

For information address BG Publishing LLC,
1619 Harbor Avenue SW, Suite 200, Seattle WA 98126.

Library of Congress Cataloging-in-Publication Data
Gralpois, Bruno.
Magnifique Inside & Out: Find Out How TRULY Beautiful You Are
By Bruno Gralpois – First Edition.

FIRST EDITION.
Copyright 2015 Bruno Gralpois
Published by Waterside Press
All rights reserved

ISBN: 978-1-941768-62-4 ebook
ISBN: 978-1-941768-63-1 print edition

Dedicated to the 'magnifique' women—who have blessed my life by showing me what real beauty is.

ACKNOWLEDGMENTS

I want to acknowledge the "magnifique" women who gave me a unique understanding and appreciation for what real beauty is: my daughter and talented actress, Anaïs Gralpois, my splendid mother and everyday role model, Josette Gralpois, my adorable twin sisters Michelle Retif and Danielle Touyre, and the joy of my life and most amazing life companion, Christine Serb. Christine was a major source of inspiration and was instrumental every step of the way. I am eternally grateful for her patience, support and many ideas since the inception of this project. I am very grateful for the insight shared by my daughter Anaïs, which proved to be particularly helpful in understanding the millennial perspective.

This book would have not been possible without the contribution of so many wonderful individuals with a shared passion for this topic:

The many well-recognized subject matter experts who have enhanced the value of the book by sharing their vast knowledge in their respective fields of study and/or practice: Susan Kleiner (nutrition), Linda Melone (fitness), Bobby Bakshi (confidence building), Robyn Hatcher (communication), Michael Fertik (reputation management) and Karen Starns (personal branding).

The remarkable women I interviewed for this book and shared their valuable secrets to success with us all: Brittney Dawn Brannon, Connor Boss, Heidi Forrest, Kristen Dalton, Marika Siewert, Maureen Francisco, Melanie Kannokada and Susie Castillo. My friend Maureen Francisco was not only a great contributor; she also offered her help and support on many occasions. Lola White and Dr. Elizabeth Lindsey offered great insight and perspective.

Justin Hebert for his remarkable photographs. Justin has a unique gift and artistic talent. He used both to create and select stunning photographs to accompany this book and make it more enjoyable to read. I want to thank David VanMauran for the pictures he generously contributed, as well as Allyson Rowe, Miss Washington USA 2014 for allowing me to use her picture in this book.

Paul Prentice and Erika Gonzalez at Prentice Design for their superb graphics design skills and much-needed creativity and art direction for the cover and the many graphics in the book. Bill Gladstone and the team at Waterfront Press for getting the book published.

My faithful friend Patricia Berns for her continuous support and encouragement, always there to offer valuable connections and ideas. My longtime friend Frederic Vimeux for his acute understanding of legal matters.

I also conducted focus groups with a number of willing participants and book aficionados who read earlier versions of the manuscript, provided great suggestions which improved the quality of this book, and for whom I am most grateful (in no particular order): Jamei Jure, Latasha Haskins, Chris Bajuk, Abigail Leonard, David Huynh, Michelle Font, Elena Tavakoli, Roxie Drofiak, Margeaux Rabbage and Yasuyo Isono.

The entire team at Penn Schoen Berland (PSB), Tammy Kaneshige, Mark Burles and Alyssa Landry for their exceptional contribution to the research we conducted on women's and men's perceptions of beauty. Special thanks to my friend Jake Sedlock, for his vision and support, going the extra mile to rally everyone at PSB behind this research project and being so committed to this topic.

Nancy Buffington for her exceptional editing skills and unique perspective that enhanced the quality of the book and made it a more enjoyable reading experience.

Finally, I am enormously grateful to my amazing son Max and to my family in France for their love and support, but also for their patience as I threw myself passionately into this book, dedicating much of my weekends to make it a reality.

BRUNO GRALPOIS

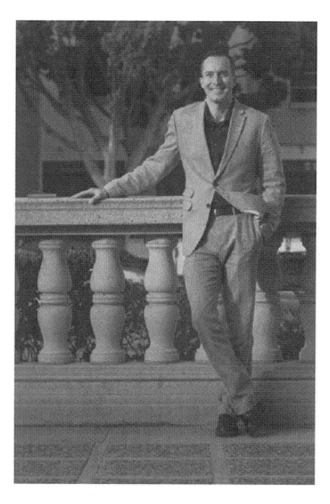

A high-profile business executive, Bruno has spent the past 20 years driving marketing and brand excellence for the world's most prestigious companies. A Microsoft veteran of 10 years, he received the prestigious Microsoft Marketing Excellence Award from former CEO Steve Ballmer for his exceptional leadership. Bruno held high-level positions at other successful Fortune 100 companies including Visa Inc. His book *Agency Mania,* now available in multiple languages, is considered a reference book in the business community. Recognized as a leading authority by his industry peers, he is a frequent speaker at industry events and is often quoted in the media. He's a French Foreign Trade Adviser for the French Ministry of Trade and Commerce. A French native, Bruno grew up near Paris, the world-renowned center of style, beauty and fashion. A pro bono adviser for two-time Academy Award® winning actress Emma Thompson and world-known fashion and portrait photographer Nick Haddow, Bruno's passion lies in protecting human rights and helping others realize their true potential.

COVER AND GRAPHIC DESIGN by Erika Gonzalez (Prentice Design, Inc., Seattle, Washington).

ORIGINAL PHOTOGRAPHS by Justin Hebert and David VanMauran.

All trademarks, copyrighted material, service marks and other registered materials used herein remain the lawful property of their rightful owners.

Visit our website at: www.magnifiqueinsideout.com

Waterfront Press and BG Publishing

MAGNIFIQUE

INSIDE & OUT

Find out How TRULY Beautiful You Are

TABLE OF CONTENTS

INTRODUCTION

La vie est belle (life is beautiful), the French like to say. But for those of us who don't live comfortably nestled in the charming Riviera town of St. Tropez, life can seem challenging, even unfair. Being a woman in today's youth-and-beauty-obsessed society is increasingly stressful. Women must compete—with other equally ambitious individuals—for the best grades, schools, jobs and relationships. In today's world, nothing is a given; everything must be earned. It's no wonder that many women wake up each day feeling like they're onstage and everyone is keeping score! No matter her ethnicity, age, economic background, family status, profession or personal connections, today's woman faces a daunting but inescapable task: she must apply herself thoroughly, put forward the best version of herself and work hard to cross every finish line victorious. It is a race, no doubt ... and the race is well underway.

For one woman, it might be a soul-searching journey: discovering who she is, following a vocation, learning to feel comfortable in her own skin or chasing a lifelong dream. For another, it might be finding the right partner, building a family, pursuing a new profession, climbing a career ladder or mastering a difficult craft. The struggle for personal and professional success is a mirror for the complicated, often conflicting challenges faced by an entire generation of women. Even the signature song of legendary French cabaret singer Édith Piaf, *"La Vie En Rose"* (which translates as "Life Through Rose-Colored Glasses"), provides little comfort to those looking for real answers. The only way out of this downward spiral is to face that mirror, understand its origin, and deal openly with it. And to heed the warning on every car's side mirror: objects in the mirror are always closer than they appear.

If you walked into a room today filled with 25 women, how many of them do you think find themselves attractive? One. That's right, only one. This is not fiction or an isolated phenomenon either. The large majority of women fail to find themselves beautiful—and we have grown accustomed to this sad reality. If you're reading this book, chances are good that you might be inclined to feel that way. This shocking finding demonstrates why there are no greater obsessions in today's society than beauty and the endless pursuit of physical perfection. Women today feel more pressure than ever to look their very best, at home and in their work space. Conditioned by popular culture and mass media, women of all ages and ethnicities—all around the world—obsess and struggle over their appearance, starting at a very young age. They invest an incredible amount of time, energy and money hoping to conform to today's narrow definition of beauty, often missing opportunities to pursue other superb, less physical expressions of beauty.

As social creatures, we're naturally influenced by society and media outlets. As consumers, we're bombarded daily with retouched images of supermodels with flawless skin, lustrous hair, sculpted muscles and more, beckoning to us from billboards and commercials alike. Which means that, as individuals, we find ourselves pressured and conflicted. These consumer images serve as painful reminders of the often-unattainable standards of beauty that have contributed for decades to women's low levels of confidence and self-esteem. To reverse this dangerous trend, women must cultivate more than good looks to regain confidence and find real happiness. They need to reclaim the true meaning of beauty—inside *and* out–and make it more than a remote fantasy.

Initiation to the Beauty Industry

I was born in Nantes, France, in the Northwest region. Nantes is near Paris, the world's renowned capital of love and beauty, and the birthplace of countless premier fashion houses: Chanel, Dior, Givenchy, Jean-Paul Gaultier, Hermès, Louis Vuitton, Yves Saint Laurent and many others whose creations fill the dazzling store windows of the Avenue des Champs-Élysées.

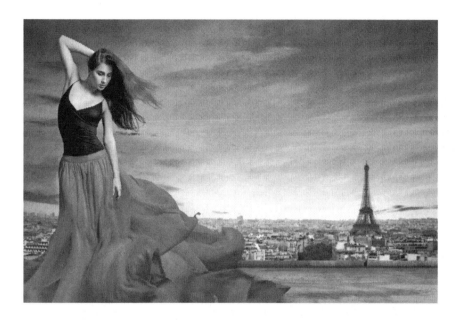

The world I came from has been known for centuries to celebrate artful expressions of the beautiful—the *magnifique* which in French means "magnificent" or "marvelous." The French seem to have considered themselves beauty experts since the dawn of time. Countless sculptors, painters and artists from the old continent have dedicated their lives to capture female beauty in ways both graceful and expressive. The Greek sculpture Venus de Milo, believed to depict Aphrodite, the Greek goddess of love and beauty, is a powerful reminder of our passion for beauty. Not surprisingly, you can find the famous sculpture on the Right Bank of the Seine in the 1st *arrondissement,* in the renowned Louvre Museum in Paris.

Beauty still occupies a privileged place in the French national identity and vocabulary, on par with its exquisite food and wine. A product of my environment, I learned at a young age to appreciate people who took great pleasure in offering the best physical and artistic expressions of themselves to the world.

My epiphany really happened a few decades later and thousands of miles away from my native home, with an invitation to join a panel of local celebrity judges, as a best-selling author and business executive, for the Donald J. Trump and NBCUniversal joint venture Miss Washington USA® pageant. Although the world of beauty contests—in Europe or the U.S.—was largely a mystery to me, I accepted that invitation with a curious and open mind. My experience in the business world, holding leadership marketing positions at prestigious companies like Microsoft and Visa, taught me to spot talent quickly. It also gave me a unique appreciation for how individuals can apply common-sense marketing and branding principles to build and successfully project an authentic, inspiring image of themselves to others. I would make use of these competencies, in partnership with other judges, to recognize the most promising candidates.

I was well aware of the pageant industry's reputation for being superficial. The cynical among us would suggest that these events promote beauty icons more concerned with the fit of an evening gown than a charismatic personality, moral sensitivity or professional accomplishments. I was nevertheless intrigued by the genuine commitment of these women to devote an entire year of their lives preparing for a rewarding—yet demanding—human endeavor that most of us wouldn't dare contemplate. Through their life experiences and a commitment to something bigger than themselves, they would come to challenge a wealth of common stereotypes, along with my own preconceived notions of the meaning of beauty.

What I discovered was a community of gifted, humble, inspiring, caring women—each of them eager to face a world of tremendous potential. They were not alone. Over the following years, I met remarkable leaders and splendid individuals who pursued stellar careers and personal dreams. I didn't see it at first, but I came to realize that they all had something special in common: they all had overcome extraordinary life challenges that set them apart. They were beautiful to the eye and heart alike. But in my view, they shared something even more amazing: a vision for a better, more fulfilling definition of beauty in our society.

We see many remarkable women with stunning figures as strikingly beautiful—but for all the wrong reasons. We—and they— must learn how truly beautiful they are, for reasons that have nothing to do with their genetic predispositions or the personal circumstances of their past. It is their inspiring stories of survival and commitment to others—stories which often garner far less media attention—that make them truly *magnifique.*

Beyond Physical Appearance

As I interviewed successful women about the secrets to real, fulfilling beauty, I felt privileged to meet the next generation of female leaders and role models: talented women showing great potential, passion and perseverance in facing enormous challenges. They exhibited a remarkable mix of mental discipline, emotional strength, memorable personalities, impeccable reputations and healthy lifestyles. You are about to learn their secrets in this book.

The women I interviewed over the years, whether contestants, judges or successful professionals with no connection with the beauty industry, invited me to look at the world differently. They offered a more just and promising future for women. These women defied the stereotypical image of shallow beauties who exploit their appearance as their sole asset. They radically changed my perspective, and I suspect they might change yours too. They had begun a "voyage" that truly changed their lives: one that strengthened them physically, mentally, emotionally and spiritually, and prepared them for a bright future full of new opportunities.

Even in a world that portrays female beauty as neither attainable nor satisfying, going beyond external attributes and embracing the idea of *inner* beauty can help any woman live a more satisfied life. These women had learned much about themselves from coaches, mentors, experts and each other; they were well underway in their personal journeys to building character and self-confidence. They applied this new understanding of "true" beauty in their everyday lives, starting companies and new ventures, organizing fundraisers, negotiating business deals, leading public debates and giving back to their communities.

Learning from Others

As I listened to this array of accomplished women reveal their personal dreams, commitment to social issues, and desire to become voices for those less fortunate, I realized that their experiences could benefit others, on a much larger scale.

Authentic, empowering experiences had given them access to valuable knowledge and resources not otherwise available to them, and completely unavailable to the general public. Could we offer others the opportunity to learn the secrets of well-being, happiness and self-esteem that had transformed these remarkable women? Could any woman apply these sensible lessons to better herself? Will we finally decipher the code of being *"magnifique* inside & out"* and make it accessible to all? The answer was easy: *Mais oui,* we ought to try!

And so I embarked on this expedition, leveraging my professional experience in storytelling and brand building, keen to share the touching stories of these successful women who happened to be amazing both inside and out. My research would reveal the necessary ingredients for inner beauty and personal success.

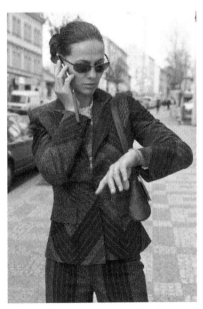

I did not go on this journey alone, by any means. I reached out to many celebrities and talented professionals in the worlds of business, media, entertainment and fashion. I enlisted the help of top-notch industry experts in nutrition, fitness, communication, confidence-building, personal branding, reputation management and many other critical disciplines to turn this book into a practical guide for any woman seeking something more than manufactured beauty or aesthetic clichés to propel her life forward and follow her dreams. This book includes poignant stories from role models and easy-to-follow tips that anyone can immediately put into practice.

Why a Man's Perspective?

Although I never was directly challenged by my family or friends, some naturally wondered why a *man* (that would be me!) was writing a book about and for *women*. From their perspectives, I couldn't speak from experience on this topic. As a son, brother of twin sisters, husband and the "papa" of an incredible daughter, I thought I had gained a tiny bit of credibility over the years to talk about women. But what could I really know about women's complex physiological, mental or emotional conditions? My friends didn't challenge the good nature of my intentions—they had grown accustomed to my passionate and relentless pursuit of diverse personal growth and human rights agendas. But clearly I could never be in the position to decipher the complex nuances and characteristics of a woman's psyche.

During the initial phase of my research, I asked myself the same question: could I really write about women and provide them purposeful insight on this complicated topic? I then discovered something fascinating from the talented women I spoke to: being a man writing about and for women actually gave me a valuable and unique perspective. To them, I was totally unbiased; I could look at the topic objectively, from the outside in. I could rely on the voices and opinions of the many women I interviewed, without applying their own filters to the stories. This made me an observer, a sort of objective and less-threatening researcher, focused on facts and data. I would go further and expand my understanding of recent trends and opinions by conducting my own independent study with a top research firm, Penn Schoen Berland. The data would provide a better perspective about women's perceptions of beauty as well as men's.

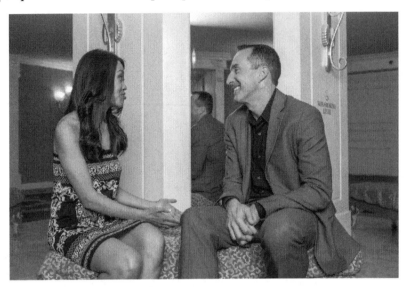

I also realized that women were more open to hearing from an "outsider," especially on a topic that is so strongly influenced by men's perceptions of women. I could provide a man's perspective on a topic commonly restricted to women's debates and conversations. I could open a conversation about our preconceived notions about what men think about female beauty, back it up with research data and invite women to reexamine their own fears and pre-conceived ideas. And these findings could give them hope.

An Open Invitation

I think you'll agree when I say that it's about time women of all backgrounds, ethnicities and origins find out or rediscover how REALLY beautiful they are. The world has never been hungrier for bright, ambitious, hardworking women who embrace change and new ideals to become much-needed leaders in business, sports, community service, and in virtually every industry that exists. By pursuing inner beauty, women are profoundly changing themselves and society's (and men's) perceptions of beauty itself.

You are not alone. No matter your background or personal or professional aspirations, I invite you to join others and take this journey yourself. I hope the stories in this book inspire you to consider a more nuanced concept of beauty—one that goes far deeper than assessing your looks in the mirror or dedicating too much precious time and money pursuing mere physical perfection. Open your mind to a new approach to reveal your authentic self—you will feel *bien dans votre peau* ("at ease with yourself"), as we say in France.

I hope this book encourages you to build and strengthen confidence and self-esteem, take excellent care of your body, mind, heart and image, balance them sensibly, and follow the path that brings you the most joy and happiness. If you do, you will be well underway to realizing your wildest, most ambitious dreams and help those around you. This book gives you the resources you need to change your life and wake up every day feeling energized and ready to conquer YOUR world. I hope it makes a positively striking difference in your life—and in the lives of others.

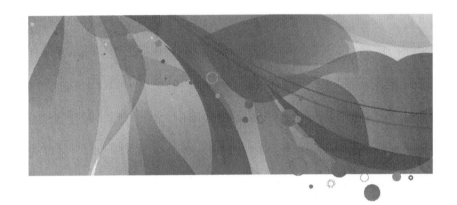

"For beautiful eyes,
look for the good in others;
for beautiful lips,
speak only words of kindness;
and for poise,
walk with the knowledge that
you are never alone."

- Audrey Hepburn
British actress and humanitarian

CHAPTER ONE

ARE WE BEAUTIFUL AND WE JUST DON'T KNOW IT?

How we feel about ourselves impacts our ability to achieve our goals. And how we feel about ourselves shapes how we appear to the world. *The Science of Sex Appeal,* a Discovery Channel documentary, makes a compelling case that humans—men and women alike—are biologically conditioned to make ourselves as attractive as possible in order to find the perfect mate.

For women, this means accentuating what science has proven to be the most determining factors in sex appeal: facial symmetry, a shapely figure, healthy-looking skin and graceful movement. In other words, a major part of sex appeal—at least initially—comes from external beauty.

External beauty is one of the variables in "assortative mating," a nonrandom mating pattern in which individuals with similar characteristics mate with one another.

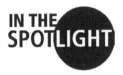

IN THE SPOTLIGHT

The Science of Sex Appeal

Are we biologically programmed to mate? Is sight the most powerful factor in our evolutionary history in determining our mate selection?

According to the Discovery Channel documentary *The Science of Sex Appeal,* chemistry is what brings us together; our choices are often more subconscious than conscious. The film explores the science of human attraction: sounds, sights and smells affect how attracted we are to each other. Genetic, hormonal and neurological factors bring people together. Our biochemical odors and voice pitch are important contributors to sex appeal. But attraction is also determined by what we see: face shape, body shape, body movement and skin.

Dr. Cara DiYanni, a psychology professor at Rider University, argues that "we are biologically predisposed to find certain aspects of humans to be attractive." She adds, "men find women with an hourglass figure to be attractive. This is partially biological in origin because wider hips signify fertility and the ability to give birth." But there's more: "Biologically, men also tend to be drawn to women with longer hair, larger breasts and healthy weights because again, these are indicators of fertility." Without these attractiveness cues (health and fertility) it would be difficult for humans to differentiate which genes are best fit to pass on to offspring.

No matter our human aspirations, can we ignore our primate instincts? Apparently, the answer is no.

We humans are very adaptive, and we instinctively understand the laws of human attractiveness. This partly explains why billions of dollars are spent each year in the fashion, cosmetic, perfume and fitness industries—just to name a few—by female (and male) consumers wanting to look their very best. Yes, many women are doing this for themselves. But they are also hoping to stand out in their personal or professional worlds by looking as attractive as possible. They want to become tomorrow's

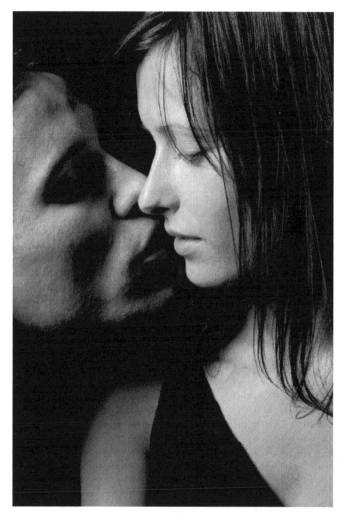

leaders, actresses, entrepreneurs, models, journalists and TV celebrities; some use their talents to advance a charitable cause and make a difference for others. They want to express themselves. They want to exhibit assertiveness. They want to find the ideal life partner. They want to impress others and leave a good impression.

No matter our goals, it's in our nature to leverage our personal assets, physical or non-physical, embrace the universal laws of attractiveness and make the best of what we have. Let's be realistic: women want to look beautiful because beauty is often associated with fame, financial success, status and power. The quest for beauty has always had a biological purpose, but our motivations often go well beyond biology.

Is There An Ugly Side of Beauty?

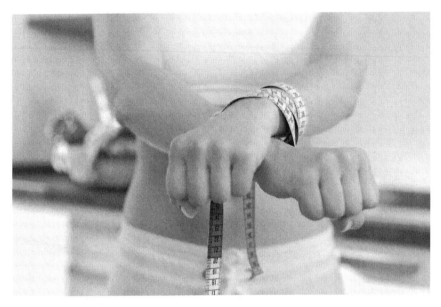

In researching this book, I asked myself this very question. Director Brent Huff asked the same thing in his 2013 documentary, *Chasing Beauty,* offering a rare glimpse into the controversial and complex world of modeling. The answer is not so surprising: our search for perfection in physical beauty has become increasingly obsessive, even destructive.

Huff's documentary goes beneath the glossy covers of fashion magazines and uncovers uncensored stories of the less-than-glamorous lives of top models and cover girls. According to the documentary:

- 25% of young American women would rather win America's Next Top Model than the Nobel Peace Prize
- 23% would rather lose the ability to read than their shapely figures.

So you may ask: is America truly obsessed with beauty? *America the Beautiful*, a documentary about self-image directed by Darryl Roberts, explores the female body image in a society dominated by unrealistic standards of beauty. Beauty is a fascination for both men and women, and a daily obsession for many. Through the use of top models—many of whom struggle with their own bodies—the billion-dollar beauty industry sells consumers a dangerous lie: greater physical beauty will improve your quality of life. Have we gone simply too far? Apparently so.

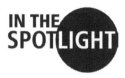

IN THE SPOTLIGHT

America the Beautiful

According to Director Darryl Roberts:

- The US has 5% of the world population but is exposed to 40% of all advertising—nowhere else are people more likely to believe that their appearance defines them
- Just three minutes looking at a fashion magazine makes 70% of women of all ages feel depressed, guilty and shameful
- The average American woman is 5'4" tall and 140 pounds; the average American model is 5'11" tall and 115 pounds
- Estimates for women "sometimes or often" on a diet: college women 91%, high school girls 40-60%, girls 9-11 years old 46%
- 9 out of 10 girls regularly use cosmetics at age 14
- American women spend $12.4 billion on cosmetic surgery and over $45 billion dollars a year on cosmetic and beauty products.

Unrealistic Standards of Beauty

A monumental mismatch exists between how we define "true beauty" and how we express it in our culture.

These undesirable labels have been powerfully communicated and amplified through the media. They have been assimilated through a culture of celebrity and an obsession with thinness and body perfection, as brilliantly captured in *Beauty Mark* another great documentary by Diane Israel, Carla Precht & Kathleen Man Gyllenhaal about self-image and the disconnect between the mind and body.

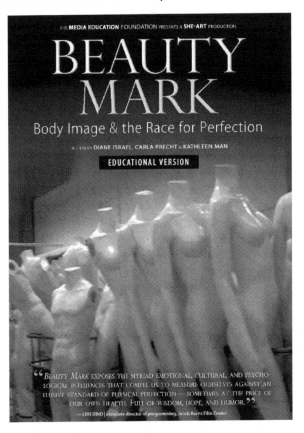

Beauty Mark exposes the myriad emotional, cultural and psychological influences that compel us to measure ourselves against an elusive standard of physical perfection—sometimes at the price of our own health. The film examines popular culture's toxic emphasis on weight through the eyes of psychotherapist and former world-class triathlete Diane Israel. An elite runner and triathlete until age 28, Israel won several major races but retired from competition after collapsing from anorexia. In the face of intense pressure to be beautiful and successful, she fell into a near-fatal spiral of disordered eating and obsessive exercising. She eventually became a psychotherapist and is now a professor of human development and a counselor, helping others deal with similar challenges.

The standard against which women measure themselves is one that is difficult (if not impossible) to achieve. This barrage of false ideas and images has been brutal for generations of young women who grew up in such a toxic social environment.

A recent global study commissioned by Dove showed that a very small percentage of women—as little as four percent—claim to feel beautiful. You read that right: only four percent! These results are deeply concerning. A majority of women believe that society expects them to enhance their physical attractiveness. Not surprisingly, 72% of girls report feeling pressure to be beautiful. In my own research, 90% of women and men in the U.S. indicated that, when it comes to beauty, women put too much focus on physical appearances; 94% believe that women are too critical of their own appearance.

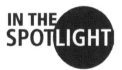
IN THE
SPOTLIGHT

"The Real Truth About Beauty"

"The Real Truth about Beauty: A Global Report" is a global study commissioned by Dove® (one of Unilever's largest Beauty Brands). The report focused on women, beauty and well-being; it made clear that it is still important to address anxieties about physical appearance.

Dove's research into self-esteem, body image and body confidence uncovered the difficulty women and girls face in recognizing their real beauty. The research confirmed that beauty-related pressure *increases* and body confidence *decreases* as girls and women age.

Key findings:
-   Only 4% of women consider themselves beautiful, a feeling shared regardless of age
-   Only 11% of girls are comfortable using the word "beautiful" to describe themselves
-   Almost half of women (47%) rate their body weight as "too high," a trend that increases with age
-   60% believe that society expects women to enhance their physical attractiveness
-   Over half of all women (57%) strongly agree that "the attributes of female beauty have become very narrowly defined in today's world"
-   More than two-thirds of women (68%) strongly agree that "the media and advertising set an unrealistic standard of beauty that most women can't ever achieve"
-   45% of women agree that "women who are more beautiful have greater opportunities in life"
-   89% believe that a woman can be beautiful at any age
-   Globally, more than half of women (54%) agree that they are their own worst beauty critics.

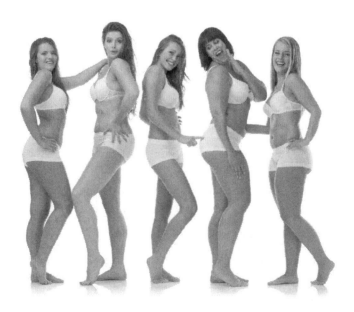

Why such pressure? In the research we conducted, 66% of respondents (men and women) agreed that beautiful women are usually more successful. So yes, beauty is still highly valued in society. Although 55% of men and women disagree that beautiful women are usually happier, especially as we get older and perhaps wiser, beauty remains an important driver of overall well-being and self-confidence. We are facing a black hole of self-esteem. How do we convince the large majority of women that they are beautiful, so they can pursue the happy, fulfilling lives they deserve?

Although studies showed that women generally hold similar views on the role of beauty, that notion of beauty has been strained by a constant barrage of physical clichés in magazine ads and TV commercials. These images have become the new norm. No wonder that this narrow, simplistic, physically focused definition of beauty makes many women conclude that they're not beautiful, and contributes to feelings of unhappiness and low self-worth at a younger age than ever before.

A few other eye-opening statistics:

- Over 60% of girls avoid certain activities because they feel bad about their looks—23% won't go to the beach or pool

- 92% of girls say they want to change at least one aspect of their physical appearance, with body weight ranking highest

- The body fat of models and actresses portrayed in the media is at least 50% less than that of healthy women.

You might wonder, as I do: what are the long-term implications on our society? The film *Miss Representation* addresses this question directly, exposing how mainstream media contributes to the underrepresentation of women in positions of power and influence in America.

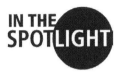
IN THE
SPOTLIGHT

Miss Representation

Miss Representation is an award-winning documentary by Jennifer Siebel Newsom that premiered at the 2011 Sundance Film Festival. Rich in interviews with Condoleezza Rice, Nancy Pelosi, Katie Couric and other leaders, the film argues that the media's disparaging portrayals of women and girls make it difficult for them to achieve leadership positions or even to feel empowered in everyday life.

Newsom exposes some shocking data:

- Although women make up just over 50% of the U.S. population, they hold only 3% of powerful positions in mainstream media
- Women hold only 20% of the seats in the House of Representatives
- Only four percent of Fortune 500 CEOs are women
- Girls between 11 and 14 see an average of 500 ads a day
- Eighty percent of 10-year-old American girls say they have been on a diet. The number-one magic wish among young girls age 11-17 is to be thinner. Fully 65% of American women and girls report disordered eating behaviors.

This is not a phenomenon limited to the United States. We've seen similar evidence in many countries around the world, from Brazil to France. Yes: even in France, the uncontested epicenter of fashion and beauty. The French television show *Beautiful Naked* goes after similar record-low self-esteem levels among French women. It does so by inviting female participants to rebuild their confidence by entirely reinventing themselves. This is an epidemic of global proportions.

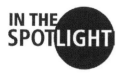

Belle Toute Nue ("Beautiful Naked")

The obsession with beauty is not merely a U.S. phenomenon, as evidenced by a popular show on French television. In France, only 14% of women report feeling good in their bodies. Too tall, too little, too heavy, too skinny—these concerns about physical appearance and lack of confidence are devastating, often preventing women from enjoying happy, fulfilling lives.

In one episode, Sylviane, 56, is self-critical, dislikes her figure and shows an utter lack of confidence. In another show, Audrey, 27, has already had cosmetic surgery twice; despite repeated efforts to improve her appearance and constant dieting, she still struggles to find herself beautiful compared to favorite celebrities.

The thought-provoking show is led by French stylist William Carnimolla, who advises "haute couture" fashion icons and French celebrities. Carnimolia invites women on the show to completely reinvent themselves, changing their image from head to toe in order to rediscover who they are and find ways to stand out.

Thankfully, there is hope: a growing number of women-led organizations and community leaders have come together to reverse these dire trends. Yet despite this sudden awareness, we still face a number of cultural phenomena that get in the way of real, sustained progress. Let's take a look at these phenomena.

Irresponsible Advertising and the Cult of Thinness

Increases in breast implants and liposuction are clear indications that the obsession with the flawless body is alive and well. It's a massive industry, worth billions to those who profit from it. But are they friends or foes? Do they contribute to a better society and healthier moms, sisters, spouses, daughters? You be the judge—by now, you probably know where I stand.

Advertising plays an important role in shaping our culture— one that goes well beyond selling products and services. I should know: I dedicated a good part of my professional life to building strong, successful brands for some of the largest companies in the world. Advertising sways consumers with the subtle argument that a particular product or service is *the* solution to a problem that perhaps they didn't even know they had. It often inspires us. It makes us laugh. It connects with us deep down emotionally. Advertising changes our perception of what is right or wrong, our expectations of family, love and even happiness.

Responsible advertising has the power to create or contribute to a healthy and socially responsible environment for consumers. But without a healthy dose of self-regulation or morality, it can also create a poisonous environment, conditioning women to believe that a certain look is all they need to find success and happiness. And all too often, this is what happens.

Whenever advertising promotes unrealistic standards of beauty or unhealthy images of women, it contributes to a negative perception of women in general, to objectification (the treatment of women as a commodity, object or instrument of sexual pleasure) and even violence.

In *Killing Us Softly,* a documentary about the impact of sexist and misogynistic images and messages, Jean Kilbourne demonstrates the negative consequences of careless advertising. The film offers a thought-provoking and inspiring look at advertising through an analysis of hundreds of print and television ads inviting women to spend money and energy in pursuit of physical perfection. Kilbourne uncovers a steady stream of sexist and misogynistic images and messages, exposing a devastating pattern of gender stereotypes and a world of frighteningly thin women in passive, dehumanizing positions that undermine girls and women in the real world.

In recent years, digital alteration has gone way too far. The clever and highly acclaimed advertising campaign launched by Unilever as part of its Dove® Campaign "Evolution" illustrates how our notion of beauty can be distorted by digitally manipulating images and tricking consumers to see what is not. The spot opens with a woman wearing no makeup, acting as a model for a new billboard advertisement. She works with a makeup

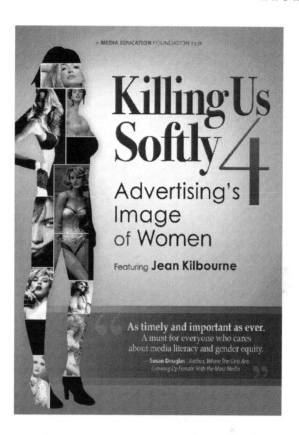

artist to change her physical appearance and mask her slight "imperfections." The fast-moving video tracks rapid changes to the model's face. It then moves to show digital enhancements made to her photos using a generic image-editing software: lengthening her neck, thickening her heir, adjusting the curve of her shoulders, filling out her lips, smoothing out her skin, enlarging her eyes and narrowing her face for a close-to-perfect final product. The end result is an image of a model rendered almost unrecognizable, then transferred to a billboard advertisement for a fictional brand of foundation makeup. The spot ends with the following message: "No wonder our perception of beauty is distorted." This ad was part of the company's efforts to free women from low self-esteem issues resulting from comparing themselves to unreal images, to encourage self-acceptance and to embrace real, unaltered beauty.

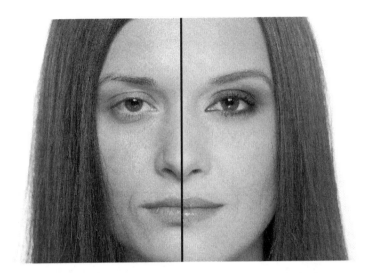

These false images of beauty objectify women in the process. Some promote products that claim to slow down or even stop the aging process—which they portray as highly undesirable. Women in ads are often pictured looking vulnerable yet suggestive, selling products from designer jeans to Skinnygirl® cocktails to Victoria's Secret® lingerie-even cheeseburgers and sandwiches like the Southwest Patty Melt in Carl's Jr. Commercials. Models are typically young women, with little-to-no consideration given to the target audience's demographics. Some ads don't even bother to display the actual product, focusing solely on the image's sex appeal to grab the consumer's attention.

There may be nothing inherently wrong with using a moderate amount of sensuality in advertising. But we can no longer pretend that they have no effect on generations of young women when an over-emphasis of superficial qualities is combined with an exclusion of other important human qualities such as confidence, sensitivity and character. Magazines and tabloids with headlines like "Pressure to be thin" or "How they get thin fast!" consistently mock celebrities who have gained weight, suggesting that success and thinness are inseparable.

Some progressive companies like H&M are taking a different approach to combat the cult of thinness, using more normal-sized models that presumably better connect with average consumers.

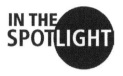
IN THE
SPOTLIGHT

H&M's Beachwear Ad Campaign

In a move to better connect with consumers and illustrate its swim-wear collection in a new and inspiring way, H&M won raves for having a "healthy-looking" woman model its beachwear after years of ads featuring unhealthily thin models. Realizing that a large part of their audience doesn't identify with size 2 models and, as a result, may not find their collection appealing, H&M selected a size 12 model to reflect a more typical American size and shape.

The public reaction on blogs was immediate, and mostly positive. Many loved that H&M had embraced "a more normal sized model" based on today's American standards, with a higher percentage of body fat.

The campaign started a debate about what is healthy or unhealthy, overweight or not, and about what perpetuates stereotypes and body shaming. Questions that emerged: what is "average" these days? If size 2 is too skinny, is size 12 too extreme or too voluptuous? How about in-between models, size 6-10? Are Americans merely looking for justifications for being overweight? Are we setting the wrong standards by showing larger-size models? Are BMI (body mass index) or body composition (lean mass ratio or body fat percentage) the only reliable criteria for determining someone's health?

No matter how we answer these questions, H&M's approach questioned the assumption that the only attractive body is a skinny one, encouraged others to recognize healthy beauty in all sizes, and showcased a larger spectrum of feminine beauty. "Normal" can be seen in every shape and size. By celebrating diverse sizing in clothing ads from mainstream companies, we open the door for a host of healthy conversations.

But look around and you'll quickly realize that companies promoting healthy standards are the exception. More often than not, images are systematically altered to promote a false image of reality. When a model is not considered slim enough, we use Photoshop to make her look thinner.

Rarely is this practice questioned. But when it is, we pay attention. Talented actress Kate Winslet was put on a diet of sorts when *GQ* magazine digitally enhanced her photograph to make her look thinner. She fought back, set the record straight about who she is and who she is *not*. Kate's actions set new standards for celebrities and every woman to follow.

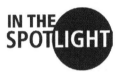

IN THE SPOTLIGHT

Kate Winslet and the GQ Incident

Kate Winslet is considered one of the most successful actresses of recent years, and a role model for many. The *Titanic* star and Golden Globe and Academy Award winner is one of the few movie celebrities refusing to allow the media to dictate her weight or conform to Hollywood's beauty standards. Or to even allow art departments to retouch her pictures before publication.

When the British *GQ* magazine put Kate on a virtual diet by digitally enhancing her photograph without her consent, she issued a statement saying, *"I don't look like that, and, more importantly, I don't desire to look like that. I can tell you they've reduced the size of my legs by about a third."*

In an interview led by the *Sydney Morning Herald*, Kate insisted: *"Nobody is perfect. I just don't believe in perfection. But I do believe in saying, 'This is who I am and look at me not being perfect!' I'm proud of that."* She made it clear that she doesn't believe in artificial standards of beauty where a woman has to be a size 2 to be attractive. *"I resent that there is an image of perfection that is getting thinner and thinner,"* she added.

Kate Winslet doesn't want the public to be misled by unrealistic images or false expressions of beauty. She doesn't want her image to fuel an idea of physical beauty that simply doesn't exist.

The Culture of Celebrity

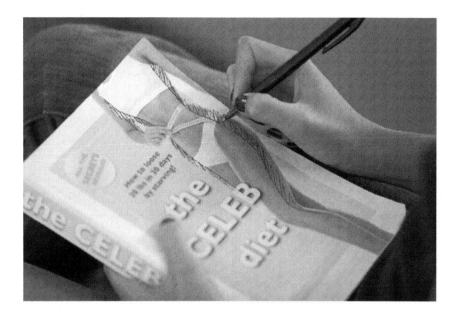

Yet advertising is not the only culprit. Does our celebrity culture have an undesirable effect on our perception of what is normal? Of course. Open a magazine or turn on the TV and you'll see celebrities and models looking like a million bucks—literally. Since our society is obsessed with physical beauty, we tend to celebrate those who fit the mold: the fit, slim, sexy and exotic. Front covers from magazines like *Women's Health, Marie Claire* or *Cosmopolitan* offer catchy headlines and inescapable tips on how to "flatten your belly," get a "bikini body now," "look great naked" or "shed one size." Sound familiar?

It's easy to forget how many stylists, hairdressers, dressmakers, fashion designers, make-up artists, stage technicians, photographers, personal coaches and fitness professionals work behind the curtains full-time to turn celebrities into the icons they're expected to be. We seem to forget that these images are as much art as anything else . . . they're rarely real human expressions of everyday life. Would we buy these magazines if they did? We obsess about superstars; we study and follow their every move: how they look, what they wear, what they eat.

Thankfully, on rare occasions, we meet personalities that stand out from the unhealthy stereotypes: women like Oprah Winfrey and Ellen DeGeneres, who offer a much-needed alternative to the endless parade of aesthetically beautiful actresses, singers and supermodels. Outspoken actress Ashley Judd challenged the media and what she considered a misogynistic attack on celebrities like herself, and ultimately women.

"Get out of My Face"

Ashley Judd is an icon of American television and films. A talented actress, she has become increasingly involved in global humanitarian efforts and political activism. Outspoken on issues she cares about, she recently made news through an eloquent response to a media frenzy regarding her supposedly "puffy face."

It all started when Judd appeared on a Canadian talk show to promote her new television series, *Missing*. Shortly after, tabloid magazines speculated that injectable fillers contributed to her puffier-than-normal face. Judd attributed her puffiness to steroids prescribed to treat a sinus infection. But what she called a "pointedly nasty, gendered and misogynistic" attack on women led to a debate about femininity in our culture. Fed up with a culture of physical objectification, she fought back waves of wild speculation about her appearance, asserting, "I do not want to give my power, my self-esteem, or my autonomy, to any person, place, or thing outside myself." Judd added, "I thus abstain from all media about myself. The only thing that matters is how I feel about myself, my personal integrity, and my relationship with my Creator."

Judd became a much-needed voice in the fight for greater dignity for women in a materialistic and misogynistic culture. She insisted, "The insanity has to stop, because as focused on me as it appears to have been, it is about all girls and women." Judd couldn't be more right. Take notice . . . and please, get out of her face!

Being Beautiful

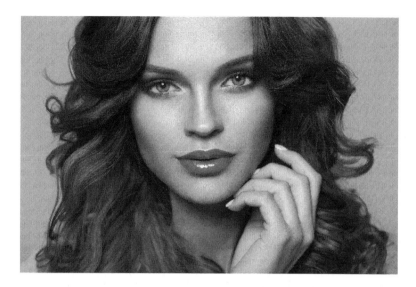

Beauty has historically been highly visual, celebrated in portraiture, sculpture and similar traditional art forms, and more recently in fashion magazines, television and beauty contests. I have come to realize that, as consumers of these eye-catching images, we all contribute to the stereotypes that support this narrow definition of beauty. When we look only at the surface, we fail to explore the multi-dimensional definitions of the beauty—and the women—we encounter.

Women are particularly tough on themselves, often failing to see what others see, as evidenced by another high-visibility video campaign. By comparing women's self-descriptions to those of strangers, the *Real Beauty Sketches* film proves that women are far more beautiful than they think. During the course of my research, it became quickly apparent by the abundance of blog and Facebook posts that this film had touched the heart of many women who empathized with the participants.

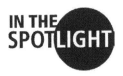

IN THE SPOTLIGHT

Real Beauty Sketches Ad Campaign

Do women see their own beauty? *Real Beauty Sketches* is a touching, provocative short film produced in 2013 as part of the Dove Campaign for Real Beauty campaign with the tagline, "You are more beautiful than you think." This eye-opening film struck a chord among women who acknowledge judging themselves too harshly.

The film set out to prove to women that they are more beautiful than they think by comparing their self-descriptions to those of strangers. Dove recruited seven women of different ages and backgrounds. Each woman described herself using "neutral and factual" terms as FBI-trained forensic sketch artist Gil Zamora, hidden behind a curtain, sketched them sight unseen. "I kind of have a fat, rounder face," said one. "My mom told me I had a big jaw," reflected another.

Earlier in the day, the women had spent time with strangers, though neither party was told why. Zamora then asked each stranger to describe the women. He created another composite sketch of each woman, this time based on the stranger's description.

The film includes emotional footage of each woman as she sees the two side-by-side sketches for the first time. The contrast between the drawings is striking: in every instance, the second sketch (based on far more positive language from strangers) is markedly more flattering than the first.

Going viral within days, it enjoyed just short of 30 million downloads and 660,000 Facebook shares during its first ten days. While media reaction was mixed, with some critics arguing that the film was too focused on appearance, an article about the campaign was shared more than 500,000 times in 24 hours.

How women approach the idea of beauty varies significantly. Some choose to develop only their professional or personal skills, refusing to concern themselves with their physical image or how they appear to the outside world. We sometimes cheer those who go "au-natural." Others choose to focus solely on improving their physical appearance, failing to develop the intellectual and emotional skills of a well-rounded person. Women are often unfairly labeled and divided into two camps: the smart, geeky (and less feminine) type, or the sensory, attractive (and less cerebral) type. Why should you be forced to choose, bowing under the pressure of a culture reluctant to grant you both? It's in your hands: you can strengthen and nurture both sides, enjoy your femininity and sensuality without compromising intellectual pursuits and personal development.

What can we do about a phenomenon that affects each and every one of us? As I began my research, it occurred to me that the cure for our misperceptions and false conditioning might lie in what might seem the most unlikely place of all. How ironic that it would be where the most physically attractive women gather that other, deeper forms of beauty would spring into life! Physical beauty would not automatically disqualify a woman from the chance to develop her heart, mind, soul and image—and the reverse would be true as well.

I would devote myself to finding the rare "magnifique" women who embrace both traditional and modern definitions of beauty, and learn how they reconcile the two. How would they manage to find the right balance? What would we learn from it? For the purpose of my research, these women would embody the most complete expression of true beauty: not by merely *looking* beautiful, but *being* beautiful as well. Magnifique, inside *and* out.

A New Definition for Beauty?

A burning need exists for a new, wider, better definition of true beauty. We know intrinsically that splendor can be found in happiness, kindness, wisdom, humor, moral sensitivity, defiance, dedication, cheer motivation and self-confidence. It can be found in simply being oneself.

The Underarmour "I Will What I Want" campaign shares stories of women athletes who overcame amazing challenges to pursue their dreams, no matter their personal situation—among them, a ballerina who didn't fit the mold by ballet standards but yet is now a soloist for the American Ballet Theatre. How inspirational!

Because not enough girls are encouraged to pursue their love of science, technology engineering and math (STEM), the 2014 #InspireHerMind Verizon campaign suggests we reverse the trend by inspiring girls to pursue high-tech jobs or join communities like Girls Who Code. 66% of 4th grade girls say they like science and math, but only 18% of all college engineering majors are female. Women hold less than 25% of our country's STEM jobs, yet 80% of jobs in the next decade will require technology skills. "Isn't it time we told her that she's <u>pretty</u> brilliant too?" asks Verizon. More than ever.

How we choose to approach and celebrate beauty is likely to affect our identity as a nation, our self-worth as individuals and, in the end, our potential as human beings. Real beauty is about being healthy: physically, mentally, intellectually, spiritually and emotionally. We are seeing renewed interest in the media and our culture for nurturing inner beauty through self-discovery, personal development, character building, perseverance and self-discipline.

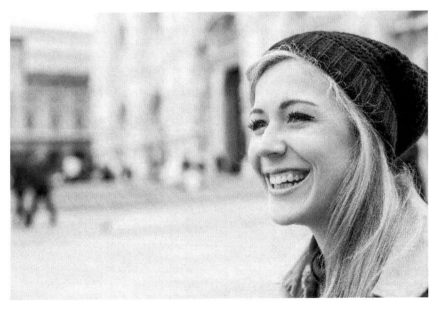

Our perception is slowly shifting; thankfully, the growth of technology and digital media has contributed to a new, broader definition of beauty as the interactive nature of today's media allows people to focus more on substance and content than on form alone. This is in clear contrast to traditional media like print or billboards that have historically fostered a more visual, static expression of beauty. In a film called *The Beauty Inside* Hollywood's first social film of its kind, interactive storytelling invites us to discover the beauty within all of us. Technology can allow us to encounter and experience beauty differently, multi-dimensionally. Real beauty can be heard and felt—not just seen. Real beauty is increasingly dynamic and fluid.

In Bare Escentuals' ad campaign "Be a force of beauty," the cosmetic company casts its women models based on who they are as individuals. The message underlying this innovative approach is equally powerful: "Pretty gets your attention. Beauty captures your heart." They couldn't have said it any better.

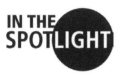

IN THE SPOTLIGHT

Be a Force of Beauty Advertising Campaign

How do you find beauty in a sea of pretty? Introducing the bareMinerals® casting story, a new campaign from cosmetics company Bare Escentuals aimed at redefining beauty. *"Pretty can turn heads but beauty can change the world. Pretty is what you are. Beauty is what you do with it,"* says an actress in the commercial. Based on the *"Be a Force of Beauty"* theme, this was the company's first-ever global creative campaign.

Bare Escentuals took a unique, personality-driven approach to casting models for TV, print and digital ads. Without seeing a single face, the company cast women who shared values with their brand, but whose beauty became palpable through their personality, compassion,

---

inspiration, honesty and confidence. The blind casting began with a survey sent to women models ages 20 to 60, asking who they were and what they were like. The company received 271 responses with stories about applicants' passions, interests and community involvement. It conducted 78 interviews and selected five who made the final cut—all without ever seeing their faces. Finalists included a volunteer firefighter and an environmental scientist.

Instead of looking, Bare Escentuals *listened.* Remaining true to their message to the very end, they allowed no retouch or airbrush photographs in the final images.

The idea behind all this work is not an empty promise to change the world overnight: irresponsible advertising, gender bias, the culture of celebrity and cult of thinness won't disappear miraculously.

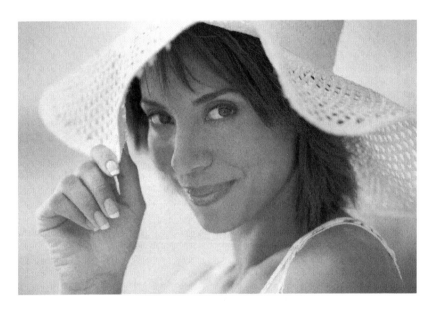

Women around the world would agree: being "Magnifique inside & out" is about pursuing ways to realize your true potential and person-hood. It means starting with your own world, one step at a time. It's about celebrating small success stories that create paths for others to follow and give millions hope that we can shape—even transform—our society for the better.

This journey is the daring union of the mind, the heart, the image and the body—in peace and harmony, glowing through from the inside out. It's a journey accessible to us all: no matter our circumstances, we can all approach life in a more balanced way, looking and feeling our best in every situation, building inner strength while doing good to others. This is the only truly worthwhile pursuit, isn't it?

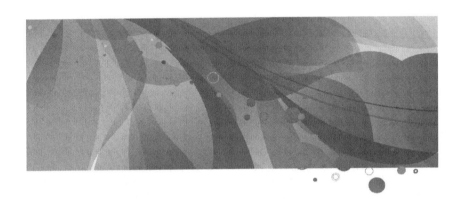

*"Everyone is like a butterfly, they start out
ugly and awkward and they morph into beautiful
graceful butterflies that everyone loves"*

- Drew Barrymore
American actress, film director, screenwriter, producer and model

CHAPTER TWO

THE PEARL IN ALL OF US

Pearls are wonders of nature. They are often used as a metaphor for something rare, fine and extremely valuable. Pearls form inside oysters, layer upon layer. It takes them years to develop and reach their peak of balance and strength. What is fascinating about the pearl's growth is its similarity to the way a woman develops natural beauty. Every woman is a pearl—or a butterfly, as Drew Barrymore puts it—at birth. Few will reveal themselves and their splendor to the world; most will hide inside their shells, uncertain of what lies beyond. Those who break free can be seen and loved for who they are: splendid and unique in every way.

Let me introduce you to some of the spectacular pearls I have been lucky enough to meet, and who share their secrets to cultivating beauty inside and out throughout this book. They include:

- a ballet dancer who reinvented herself as a TV phenomenon
- a woman with a hereditary eye disease and a remarkable will to overcome her personal circumstances
- a committed young actress who fought to stay out of homeless shelters and later became a spokesperson for the American Heart Association
- a Miss USA title owner who raised funds for breast and ovarian cancer education and research
- a Canadian recording artist who started her own record label to help artists keep their authentic voices
- a Philippine immigrant who learned English at age five and became a TV reporter and an accomplished author

- a talented bilingual TV host who grew up without a dad and overcame life challenges to become an actress, model and author
- a Stanford University graduate and former McKinsey & Company analyst, now a fast-rising Hollywood actress and co-founder of a non-profit that built a hospital in India.

When I first met these women, I couldn't help but notice how they took care to present the absolute best physical expression of themselves to the outside world. You would too, if you met them for the first time. You may also notice that some of them have participated in a beauty contest at some point. But it's not their looks or how they chose to express their external beauty I want to emphasize in this book. This is not why I picked them. On the contrary: it is their remarkable stories of defiance and courage that make these women as beautiful to the heart as they are to the eye . . . and yes, these women happen to be both. Don't under-estimate what it took them to get to this place. You can't help but notice that they're incredibly friendly, caring, determined, engaged—and yet also take pride and pleasure in taking care of their appearance. They each found a perfect balance, allowing inner and outer beauty to co-exist, and it simply shines through when they enter your life.

How do they do it? How do they balance it all? I carefully chose these inspirational, *magnifique* women, who embrace inner and outer beauty, to share their unique perspectives and words of wisdom. They will accompany us throughout the rest of the book.

Let's meet them!

Meet Brittany Dawn Brannon

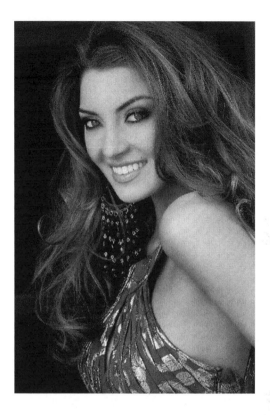

Born and raised in Scottsdale, Arizona, Brittany Dawn Brannon enrolled in classical ballet at the age of two. She pursued a passion for dancing that lasted years but came to a tragic close. Accepted to the America Ballet Theatre in New York City when she was 17, Brannon experienced a foot injury—followed by an unsuccessful surgery—that ended her promising career in ballet. She would never be able to dance again.

For Brannon, this was more than just a setback. Dancing was her life-long dream; almost overnight it was permanently destroyed. Thankfully, she had many other interests. She had studied classical violin and piano since she was five; she later joined the Phoenix Symphony Guild. She studied English Literature at Oxford and Cambridge in England, studied art in Italy and traveled the world.

> "I started ballet at age 2. I remember
> dancing fifty hours a week to become
> a ballerina. I worked so hard at it.
> After my foot surgery, I knew I would
> never dance again. It was all taken
> in an instant. One door closed but
> another one opened. I decided to enter
> my first pageant and my life truly
> changed after that."
>
> - Brittany Dawn Brannon

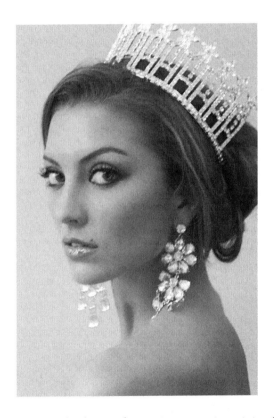

By age 21, Brannon had visited over 25 countries, giving her a unique understanding and appreciation for diverse cultures. She graduated from Pepperdine University with a major in Broadcast News and Art History.

Brannon challenged herself once more by entering the Miss Arizona USA competition—she won the title on her third attempt in 2011. Later, her natural ability to connect with others led her to positions at NBC Universal's *The Today Show* and *Nightly News*. Having found her true calling, she became the TV host for *Phoenix Fashion Week* and *Fox Sports*.

> *"Being beautiful inside out starts with the heart shining through. You are beautiful inside when you use beauty for good and invest in others."*
>
> - *Brittany Dawn Brannon*

As a leader and role model in the community, Brannon used her growing influence to help people from many backgrounds, from high school girls to veterans. To Brannon, helping others realize their dreams is an important part of what she calls real success.

Meet Connor Boss

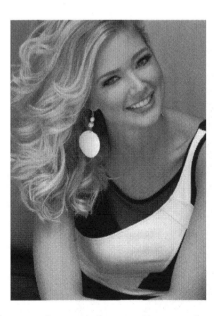

Connor Boss is a hero in the eyes of many. At just eight years old, Boss was diagnosed with a hereditary eye disease that causes progressive vision loss.

Glasses failed to improve her deteriorating eyesight, but Boss had a crystal-clear vision for her direction in life. Her peripheral vision allowed her to read enlarged computer screens and large-print textbooks at school. She sometimes ran into things and had trouble focusing straight ahead. Yet Boss turned out to be a stellar student with excellent grades; she refused special treatment and insisted on being considered on equal footing with others.

In 2012, Boss became the Miss USA pageant's first legally blind contestant. The world caught a glimpse of who she really is: a confident, funny, beautiful woman with a kind spirit and a gift for public speaking.

> *"Success is the product of passion, determination and drive. It is the incredible sensation of seeing your hard work actually pay off and bring you closer to achieving your dream."*
>
> *- Connor Boss*

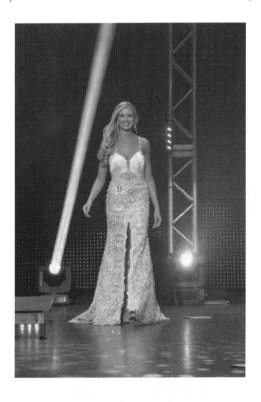

Boss's early success encouraged her to take good care of her health; this prepared her for higher-stakes competitions. At one event her weak depth perception made her stumble on stage, yet she won second runner-up as Teen Miss Florida USA. Boss's remarkable story of perseverance was picked up by major news networks from CNN to ABC News, and she became an inspiration to many.

Boss may not have won every crown—and naturally she can't drive a car. She knows she has to compensate for her poor eyesight to be success-ful. But she's an incredible role model for many with disabilities, inspiring them to overcome challenges with confidence and determination.

"The most common misconception today is to confuse beauty with pleasing physical fea-tures and sex appeal. Being beautiful inside out means so much more than this simplistic view. It is the willingness to be open to the world and a choice all women must make to shine through and from within."

- Connor Boss

Meet Heidi Forrest

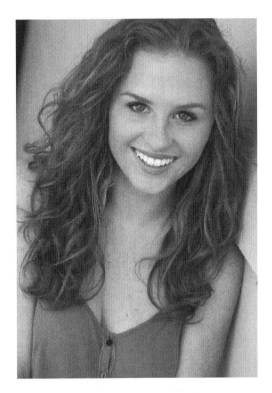

As long as Heidi Kathryn Forrest can remember, she has been a creative spirit with a passion for the arts. Like many girls her age, she wanted to be an actress.

Forrest was raised in a small town in Georgia, far from the world of entertainment that captivated her. At age 10, she had her first role in a school play; at 12 she was discovered by a talent agency and made her first commercial. She eventually convinced her mother to move to Los Angeles where she could pursue her dreams. She enrolled at Beverly Hills High School and took on many roles: varsity cheerleader, peer counselor and founder/president of school programs.

Although Forrest attended a prestigious school, she and her mother struggled financially throughout her high school years—a car accident had left her mother with severe neck and back injuries that kept her from working. Forrest walked or biked to school while her classmates arrived in expensive and exotic cars, driven by chauffeurs. Then Forrest's stepfather was diagnosed with lung cancer and lymphoma. Forrest and her mother were eventually evicted from their apartment, with shelters as their last option. Luckily, one of Forrest's friends opened her doors, offering a home until she graduated.

> *"Beauty lies within and ultimately shows through your essence. To me, a caring individual who lets her actions speak louder than her words is truly beautiful."*
>
> *- Heidi Forrest*

Not longer after, Forrest's mother experienced heart failure and needed surgery. Forrest started a fundraiser to raise awareness for heart disease and promote healthy living. Her goodwill pilot fundraiser was a huge success—it has become an annual national fundraiser for the American Heart Association, where she is now a spokesperson.

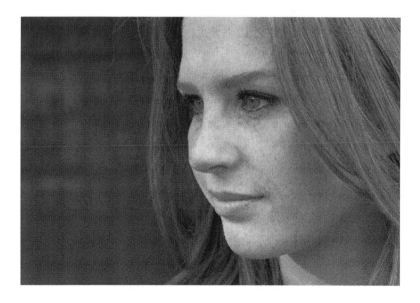

Forrest decided to pursue her childhood dream of becoming an actress. The hardships she experienced in her youth only pushed her further. She now plans to write for her own production company, creating movies that empower people to pursue their dreams regardless of circumstances. To Forrest, being beautiful is mostly about inspiring others through perseverance and genuine care for others.

> *"Being beautiful inside out means that you don't just have a pretty face and expect things in return for standing in front of a camera. It means spreading your inner beauty outward and inspiring everyone who you meet by making a difference in your community and truly caring for other people. To me, it is important today because in doing so, you are inspiring the generations of tomorrow, ultimately making a difference in human kind."*
>
> *- Heidi Forrest*

Meet Kristen Dalton

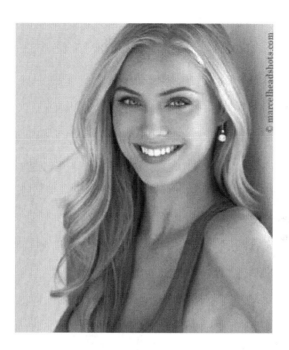

Ask Kristen Dalton and she will tell you she dreamed of becoming Miss USA since she was three years old. But growing up, Dalton never truly believed in herself; she struggled with cystic acne and body image issues. Twenty years later, her dream finally came true.

Make no mistake: Dalton didn't achieve her childhood dream by sheer luck. No matter what obstacle she faced, it was determination, preparation and a positive attitude that brought her goals within reach. By the time she received the Miss USA crown in 2009, the southern belle had become an inspiring and confident woman.

Already an accomplished singer, actress and dancer, Dalton's title propelled her to a successful career in entertainment. She is now a familiar face on TV, following her appearances on hit shows like *The Jay Leno Show, The Today Show, Good Morning America* and CNN. Dalton has also appeared in a range of commercials for Old Navy, Skechers and Allegra and is the National Spokesmodel for LA Fitness.

"Success for me is looking back in the mirror and realizing that I had a meaningful impact on people's lives. I want to know that I somehow touched people's hearts, raised them up, and helped them discover their greatness within."

- Kristen Dalton

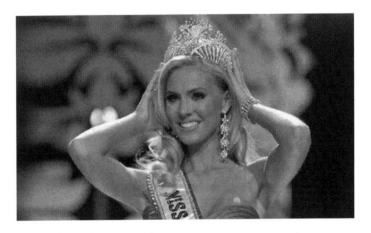

Despite her long list of accomplishments, it isn't her commercial work or modeling career that make her most proud. Her proudest moments involve encouraging girls one-on-one, being trusted to share powerful, transparent stories from women all over the world on her faith-based blog, marrying her dream husband and publishing her first devotional for girls called *Rise Up, Princess: 60 Days to Revealing Your Royal Identity*. In 2013, Kristen created the online magazine SheisMore.com, which includes devotions, inspiring stories, relationship articles, wisdom and advice reaching hundreds of thousands of women each month. Dalton's commitment to raising up confident women in their royal identity as a daughter of God through writing, speaking and mentorship is the truest expression of her beauty; her commitment has made the world more loving and more beautiful for us all.

> *"Focus on what you love, not on building a resume. I made decisions early in life to prove to the world that I wasn't just a pretty face. But at the end of the day, it doesn't matter what the world thinks - they eventually stop paying attention. What matters is your consistent joy."*
>
> *- Kristen Dalton*

Meet Marika Siewert

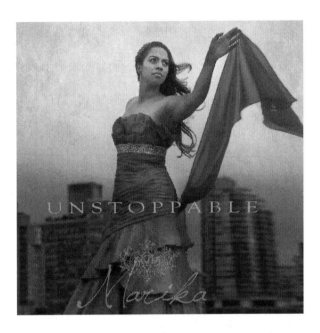

Growing up in England, she was called "Sammie" until she was 11. It wasn't until her family moved to Canada that she learned her real first name: Marika. It's by that name that the talented Canadian pop singer-songwriter is now known around the world. Siewert started playing the piano by age five, and knew early on that she wanted to devote her life to singing pop music. After countless industry accolades, Siewert garnered three top-40 singles in Canada. Her work has since been picked up by many radio, film and television venues including *America's Next Top Model*. Her songs have been aired on MTV and NBC, and her single "Angel" was featured in Lifetime Movie Network's original movie, *Sins of a Mother*. She even performed for the 2010 Winter Olympics Torch Relay, with country superstar Terri Clark. In the course of her remarkable career, Siewert has shared the stage with a range of Grammy award-winning artists.

Today, in addition to being an international singer and songwriter, Siewert is also the CEO of her own recording and production company,

Emerton Records, Inc. More importantly, she's the self-proclaimed Chief Mother Officer, a dedicated parent who leads by example and holds strong personal and family values. But it wasn't without struggles. Siewert refused to conform to standards often imposed by record labels that insist on changing an artist's appearance for commercial purposes. In an industry that is essentially image-driven, Siewert has managed to keep her music—and her appearance—truly original and authentic.

> *"I am lucky that I never had anyone to compare myself to growing up. Like everyone else, I still deal with image issues today. I think about my image, not fitting the stereotypes of other artists in the industry. My goal is to be on a global platform and encourage women in the industry to being their own self."*
>
> *- Marika Siewert*

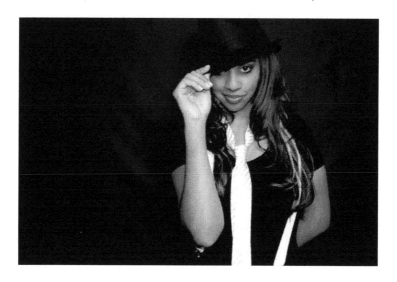

Outside the studio, Siewert works hard in organizations like "Free the Children," teen girls' confidence-building events. She's always looking to raise awareness about the need to evolve beauty standards and give back to people and communities.

Siewert continues to enjoy widespread support and recognition for her contributions to the music industry and to women in general. She started Emerton Records to stay true to her vision to change the world . . . one song at a time. She's well underway to doing just that.

Meet Maureen Francisco

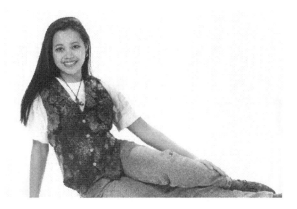

Born in the Philippines, Maureen Francisco had big dreams from the start. At age five, she moved to the U.S. with her family to pursue the American Dream. When she set foot in this country, the author of *It Takes Moxie: Off the Boat, or Out of School, To Making It Your Way in America* could hardly speak English. But Francisco would defy the odds, becoming a TV reporter and anchor after college. Always innovative, she pushed the limits of her craft: she underwent LASIK eye surgery on live TV, giving viewers a play-by-play of her experience. She was the first contestant on CBS's *Power of 10* and Fox Reality Channel *Solitary 3.0*—the highest-rated show for an original program.

> *"Women are hard on themselves. We strive to have it all and sometimes we fall below our own expectations. It's not unusual to focus on the things we don't have like beauty, relationships, etc. Yet each of us carries special beauty that no one has."*
>
> *- Maureen Francisco*

Today, Francisco is co-executive producer at NW Productions, LLC, a media and production company that produces red carpet events, reality shows and live events. Her dream: to impact millions of young people by encouraging them to fulfill their potential and realize their dreams. Francisco is also co-president of Ascend, a non-profit dedicated to boosting the leadership and business potential of Pan-Asians. She's also the executive producer of her first "docuality" (a combination of documentary and reality show) on pageant contestants who muster the courage to do things outside their comfort zones. She has been featured in, contributed to or acted as talent in more than fifty media outlets, including Forbes.com and Huffington Post.

> *"Oftentimes, people look for love, rather than being love. Beauty is what's inside. It's an ingredient found in all of us but needs to be breathed on by trusted mentors. That's why great parenting is so critical. When that happens, beauty radiates within and is an attractive and beautiful quality."*
>
> *- Maureen Francisco*

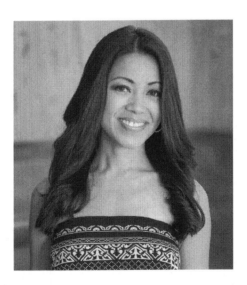

Francisco often reminds young people not to be driven by emotions; she helps them see that, by focusing on specific goals, they can accomplish great things. Fueled by courage, passion and perseverance, her life has become a remarkable American success story. Francisco clearly knows what she's talking about.

Meet Melanie Kannokada

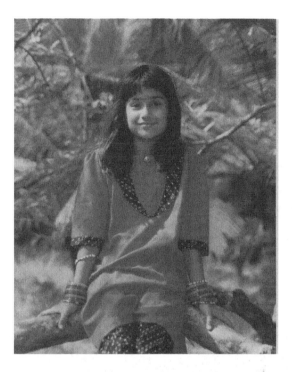

Formerly a Mechanical Engineering student at Stanford University and an analyst for McKinsey & Company, Melanie Kannokada would have become a powerful business leader—if it weren't for her deep passion for arts and entertainment.

Kannokada is not quite like anyone you've ever met before. She considers herself an actress, but she's a lot more: a techie, model, black belt in Shotokan Karate with numerous national and international victories, and a co-founder of Hospital for Hope.

Kannokada's parents moved from India to the United States. She was raised in a modest environment and learned very early on that you must work hard to get what you want in life. So she did just that, becoming a fast-rising and ambitious Hollywood actor who landed a number of high-profile opportunities.

*"I had a lot of rejections in my life.
I wanted to go to my dream school,
Stanford. I was waitlisted at first.
If I didn't fight for it, it would have
never happened. Things didn't
come easy to me. It only motivated
me to work hard at everything I
did, so no one could deny me the
opportunities I wanted to pursue."*

- Melanie Kannokada

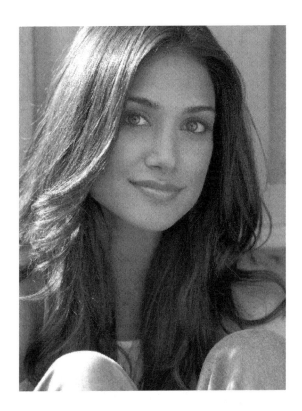

In 2011, Kannokada made her television debut with a guest-starring role on CBS's *Rules of Engagement*. She then appeared on a number of shows on ABC and NBC including *Parenthood* and *The Nine Lives of Chloe King,* and in short and feature films. She did numerous photo shoots for *Vogue* and commercials for brands like Acura, Head and Shoulders, NesCafe, Bud Light and others.

Already a familiar face on television and in print, Kannokada was chosen as one of five models by Bare Escentuals' "Be A Force of Beauty" campaign. She became the first Indian-American face of the global cosmetic brand. Despite her undeniable commercial success as a model and actress, Kannokada has committed herself to giving back to communities around the world. She's been involved in several charity events and non-profits focused on youth and education. One of her most inspiring projects: the non-profit Hospital for Hope organization she co-founded has built a self-sustainable hospital in one of the poorest states in India. The hospital provides healthcare to villagers who would otherwise have to drive three hours in good weather (twice longer during monsoon season) to get help . . . if they could afford it. Kannokada traded in her business suit and a promising career at McKinsey & Company and decided to pursue her true calling. She now focuses on acting, producing and being a brand ambassador for companies she believes in. She has become a role model for the Indian-American community and all women who want to make a difference in the lives of others.

> *"The conversation has finally begun about helping women recognize and enjoy beauty. Advertisers are catching up to this. I was lucky to be selected as one of five faces of Bare Escentuals international "Be A Force of Beauty" campaign and to be the first Indian-American to be the face of a global cosmetics brand. All five of us were selected behind a screen based on how we answered their questions, not how we looked."*
>
> *- Melanie Kannokada*

Meet Susie Castillo

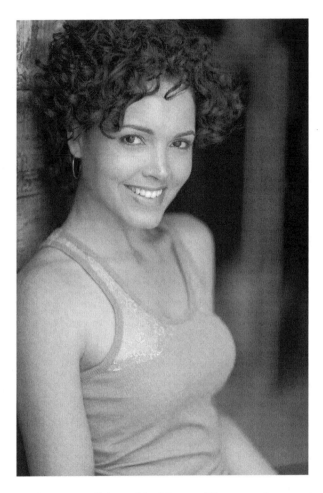

Susie Castillo likes to call herself a Ninja of Love, a plant-eating animal lover who juices veggies every day and blogs about nutrition. To the public, she has emerged as one of television's most-recognized friendly faces. Castillo is a successful bilingual TV host, actress, author, former Miss USA—and the face of Neutrogena skincare.

Of Puerto Rican and Dominican descent and fluent in Spanish, Castillo was named one of the 25 most beautiful by *People en Español*. She lives in Los Angeles with her husband and two dogs, Lupe and Oscar, pursuing a successful career in entertainment. A natural talent in life and on camera, she has been a regular host on radio and major TV networks. As an actress, she landed roles on several sitcoms and TV shows, and feature films like Disney's *Underdog*.

> *"True beauty comes from loving yourself. You can't love others if you don't love yourself. If you love the person you are, love others and live by the golden rule of treating others as you would like to be treated, then you are truly beautiful. "*
>
> *- Susie Castillo*

Castillo's dream career is to develop her own shows and entertain people with purposeful, quality content. In her inspirational book *Confidence is Queen: The Four Keys to Ultimate Beauty through Positive Thinking*, Castillo shows readers how to become confident and overcome obstacles. She draws from a wealth of personal experience: her father leaving the family when she was six, and creating a name for herself in the challenging world of entertainment.

> *"Never lose sight of who you are, no matter how successful you become. Too many women lose the sense of who they are, where they come from, how they got there and who helped them along the way. I am very appreciative of the opportunities I had in my career. I try to keep a healthy perspective on life. "*
>
> *- Susie Castillo*

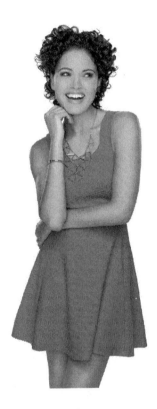

An accomplished athlete and passionate about animal welfare, Castillo spends her spare time helping non-profits and advising women about health and nutrition. She ends her voicemail message on a playful but sincere note: "Remember to eat your vegetables!" Castillo is a role model and has grown a large fan base—anyone can see why.

By now, I hope you have a better idea why I chose these *magnifique* women— Brannon, Boss, Forrest, Dalton, Siewert, Francisco, Kannokada, and Castillo—to guide us through the rest of this book. I chose role models who are beautiful to the heart but also to the eye—yes, society's most primitive expression of beauty— and have created a perfect blend of inner and outer beauty.

These women's stories reflect the importance of a healthy body, a strong mind, a confident heart and an inspiring image. They learned what it takes to find the right balance among those four qualities. They strug-gled (as we all do) and yet overcame adversity to pursue their dreams. They aspire to be the very best they can be. It's a continual journey for each of them, as it is for each of us. We are grateful for their words of wisdom.

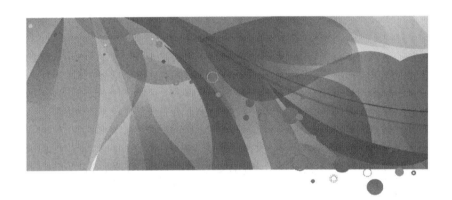

*"Though we travel the world over
to find the beautiful,
we must carry it with us
or we find it not."*

**- Ralph Waldo Emerson,
American essayist and poet**

CHAPTER THREE

RECIPE FOR SUCCESS

(When having the right ingredients is not quite good enough)

You don't need to be a Chef from Le Cordon Bleu School to know that any successful recipe requires quality ingredients: fresh produce, savory sauces, herbs and spices. But having the world's best ingredients will not guarantee a delicious dish: you also need step-by-step instructions on how to combine the right elements, at the right time.

The art and science of cultivating inner and outer beauty follow similar principles. Women have instinctive skills and abilities—and the willpower to develop them, even in the most challenging situations. Eleanor Roosevelt once said, "A woman is like a tea bag—you can't tell how strong she is until you put her in hot water." Women have the key ingredients at their fingertips to be massively successful in their personal and professional lives. But they can sometimes feel clueless about how to leverage their skills. They may not know where to start. Some—to use our cooking metaphor again—may have the recipe but lack some essential ingredients. In other words, you can't make an apple pie if you don't have apples.

> *"Success is about knowing who you are first and foremost. It's also valuing relationships over material success. The more you invest in people, the more likely you are to be truly successful."*
>
> *- Brittany Dawn Brannon*

The Right Combination of Ingredients: the BMHB Formula

In this chapter, we'll review the ingredients that are essential to success, and talk about why they matter so much. Interviews with experts from a range of fields helped me narrow the list to these few proven ingredients that are central to building a strong inner and outer shell.

> *"Success is being true to who you really are, to what your spirit really wants. Success is living your dream, whatever that dream may be. Being a mom at home or being the next Oprah. Do what makes you happy and you will be very successful."*
>
> *- Susie Castillo*

I asked Lorraine "Lola" White, a talented Personal Branding Coach, Consultant & Strategist, about what she sees as the key ingredients to success. She summarized it perfectly:

Years of experience working with successful people has given me a clear picture of what they all share in common: they enjoy what they do in life, and therefore have enough energy, love and resources to focus on career and life goals. They have strong boundaries, take extreme self-care and make time for things that are important to them. They have a belief system, they are curious and always want to take it to the next level to do better for themselves and for those lives they touch. These qualities support people to uncover the real truth about who they uniquely are and what drives them. When realized, these inner qualities burst out to reflect and emanate the beauty on through to the outside.

After years of research, I came to the conclusion that unleashing the beauty within is about finding the careful convergence of four powerful ingredients. I call this the BMHB formula:

- **B** for a healthy *body:* the amazing vehicle we depend on to move us forward and accomplish wonders

- **M** for a strong *mind:* the astonishing command center we rely on to grow wiser and more connected

- **H** for a confident *heart:* the powerful engine that fuels and energizes us, physically, emotionally and spiritually

- **B** for an inspiring *brand:* the authentic, engaging image we project to the world around us.

A Healthy Body

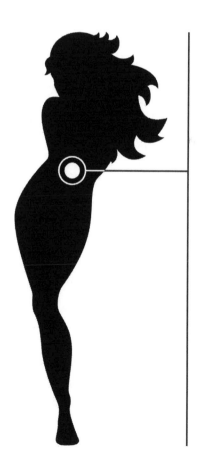

Being physically healthy is a central part of being beautiful. There's something both liberating and exhilarating about getting in the best shape of your life. You feel incredible—ready to take on life challenges with a winning attitude. But the idea of getting in great shape is often over-shadowed by the negative press around unproven weight-loss programs and questionable plastic surgeries.

We must learn to embrace diverse looks and body types, reset our expectations, and offer new generations a more progressive, more contemporary definition of beauty. Being fit and enjoying a healthy lifestyle is indispensable. It requires a combination of responsible eating, regular exercise, sufficient rest and sleep, and thoughtful skin care—all fundamental habits to shaping a healthy, beautiful body.

It *doesn't*, however, imply that women must fit a particular type, or meet certain weight or size requirements.

Being *"magnifique* inside & out" is about making the best possible use of the complex, powerful, yet fragile machine called your body. More importantly, it's about being and staying healthy both inside and out. Building a strong body is always a good investment of time and effort.

> *"We live in a celebrity culture which is highly influential in our everyday life. You watch a reality show, pick up a magazine. Our everyday lives are fueled by pop culture. So naturally, we are conditioned to have an opinion of what people should look like. In the end, it is a superficial definition."*
>
> *- Melanie Kannokada*

A strong and healthy body is the first critical ingredient in the BMHB formula and an important foundation to build on. Physical preparation goes beyond adopting healthy habits. It means giving yourself that extra boost and learning how to feel like a million "euros" at home and at work. In this book, we'll uncover commonsense principles and sound advice from world-renowned experts to provide that extra boost.

A Strong Mind

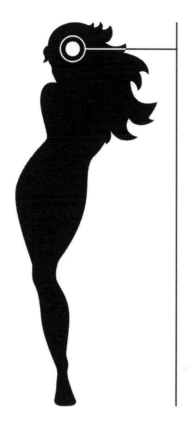

Meeting someone who, at first glance, seems remarkably attractive or charm-ing—and then turns out to lack the skills of a good conversationalist— can be very disappointing. We expect someone's "insides" to match what we see on the outside, but looks can be hugely deceiving. How can this happen?

It all starts with the brain. A remarkably intricate command center of the body, the brain is a vital organ we need to feed and nurture every day. Like any muscle, the mind needs regular exercise to develop and flourish, and to spring into action when needed. An executive may need to present results in front of a group of shareholders. An artist may need to perform in front of a large audience. A community leader may need to inspire others to take action. To really shine, each of these women must draw on skills she hones and practices every day.

Some of us are born with an innate ability to be good listeners, captivate audiences and tell engaging stories; others among us have to work hard at these skills. And our education or background varies significantly from one person to another. But our brains are sponges. We learn from each other—and from our mistakes. We are obsessively curious about everything.

> *"Beauty lies within and ultimately shows through your essence. To me, a caring individual who lets their actions speak louder than their words is truly beautiful."*
>
> *- Heidi Forrest*

A sharp, well-prepared mind helps us answer tough and unexpected questions on the spot, always landing on our feet. It helps us connect with others, ask solid, thoughtful questions and invite others into productive discussions. It helps us build our knowledge of culture, politics and world affairs. It helps us speak eloquently in private or public settings.

These are all assets that arise from a sharp mind. They make the difference between being simply noticed and being *remembered*. In this book, you will discover what successful women do to strengthen their minds and remain at their mental best in all kinds of situations.

A Confident Heart

Confidence: it's on everyone's wish list. We want to show assurance, maturity and poise in every situation. But developing confidence can a challenge. Do you walk into a room with such presence and charisma that people intuitively gravitate towards you? Do people listen carefully to your words, or do they often interrupt you? Can people easily relate to you—and can you relate to them? Do colleagues, friends or family members consistently look to you for advice?

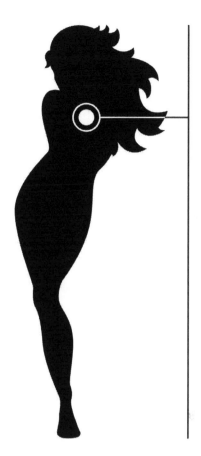

Confidence is a talent that is developed over time, when fears of rejection and failure have been conquered. It comes from the heart, which also fuels our body and mind. The heart gives us clarity about what we want to achieve, and helps us stay committed to see things through. It requires a deep understanding of our own strengths and weaknesses.

> *"I never think about life as facing challenges. I turn challenges into new opportunities."*
>
> *- Connor Boss*

To be confident means showing courage, audacity and perseverance. It is about strong character building: integrity, responsibility, risk-taking and leadership skills. In the end, confidence and emotional strength are synonyms of beauty. Being confident is an essential ingredient in a woman's success. In this book, I'll show you how to build confidence in every aspect of your life.

An Inspiring Brand

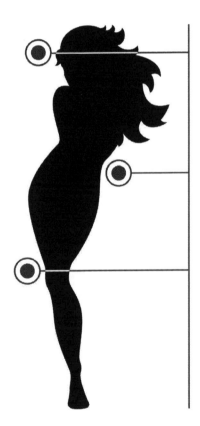

Wall Street has known all along that successful companies share one important asset: a powerful, authentic brand that makes them stand out. A reputation—whether it belongs to a company or an individual—is both incredibly powerful and surprisingly fragile. It opens doors, influences how others interact with us, and defines our values and beliefs.

A strong brand is one that stands for something unique and distinct. In business, successful brands are loved and cherished by loyal customers, and this translates into growth and profit. But people have brands too. Your personal brand impacts how people see you; it can weigh you down or significantly boost your opportunities. And its power has increased enormously thanks to technology and social media, which make information (and opinion) sharing as easy as the click of a button.

> *"There is no such thing as overnight success. When you hear about remarkable success stories, oftentimes you don't see the heartaches that came with it. Those who persevere will no doubt find success, not once or twice, but many times over."*
>
> *- Maureen Francisco*

The same principles for building and managing a brand used by companies like Nike, Coca-Cola, Starbucks or Apple apply to each of us as individuals—we are each a steward of our own brand. Think of yourself as a brand: are you truly unique, distinct and memorable? Here are some questions to ask yourself:

How do people see you?

What adjectives do they use to describe you?

Do people look up to you?

Do they follow you on Twitter or Facebook?

What do you want them to remember about you?

Is your image consistent—are you always speaking as "the same person" whether you are online or offline?

Do you come across as genuine, real and authentic?

To build and nourish a vibrant "YOU" brand requires a disciplined approach: knowing who you are, understanding how people perceive you, and creating a brand that bridges the gap between the two. It also requires a commitment to continually measure and refine your image. Overall, your personal brand should bring you closer to who you want to become. In this book, I will show you how.

What makes a woman beautiful?

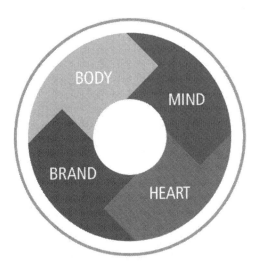

The BMHB formula involves a cohesive, holistic set of human qualities that together shape our evolving understanding of "beauty" and how it manifests in our everyday lives and our culture as a whole. When we cultivate and master all these qualities, we are truly *magnifique.*

Not only do we feel magnificent—we inspire others to follow in our footsteps. Naturally, getting there requires hard work, discipline and perseverance. We have a roadmap, but we must each take the journey in our own lives.

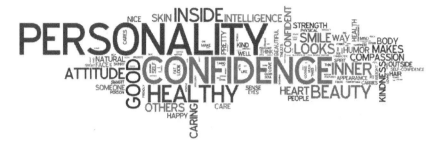

Figure 1. Word Cloud Word Cloud "What makes a woman beautiful?" (Women only)

When asked "what makes a woman beautiful?" in the study I conducted in the U.S., the answer was crystal clear as illustrated in the image above: Personality, Confidence, and Healthy were the top words respondents used in their top-of-mind responses as to what makes a woman beautiful. Generally, women believe that non-physical attributes (confidence, inner beauty) are more important than physical attributes (appearance, outer beauty).

Men and women don't all value these qualities in the same ways. When asked the open-ended question, "what makes a woman beautiful?", the majority of women favored the Heart and the Body, followed by the Brand and Mind as illustrated below.

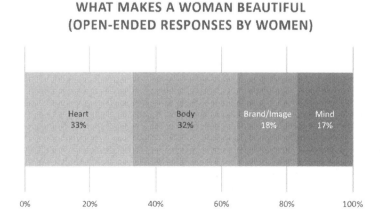

Perhaps not surprisingly, men seemed to favor the Body and Brand, followed by the Mind and the Heart.

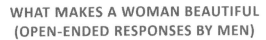
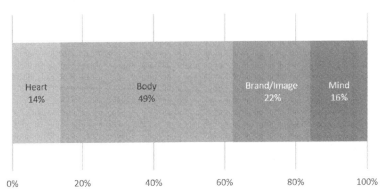

WHAT MAKES A WOMAN BEAUTIFUL (OPEN-ENDED RESPONSES BY MEN)

Heart 14%	Body 49%	Brand/Image 22%	Mind 16%

0%   20%   40%   60%   80%   100%

Looking carefully at these aggregated results for women's responses, top-of-mind responses about what truly makes a woman beautiful point to a clear choice: confidence is, by far, the most important factor. Confidence is followed closely by personality and inner self, compassion/caring and health, as illustrated below.

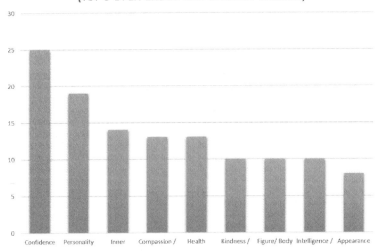

WHAT MAKES A WOMAN BEAUTIFUL (TOP 9 OPEN-ENDED RESPONSES BY WOMEN)

Men's perspective yielded interesting insights. In some ways, they validated what we might expect from men: a woman's figure/body make her beautiful. But their responses also offered some surprising, even refreshing results, as you can see below. For men, *personality* is actually what they think makes a woman beautiful, first and foremost. This is followed by a nice figure/body, valued by men far more than by most women. Men don't value "confidence" as highly as women do—but men seem to value "intelligence/education" even more than women.

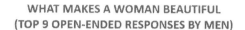

WHAT MAKES A WOMAN BEAUTIFUL
(TOP 9 OPEN-ENDED RESPONSES BY MEN)

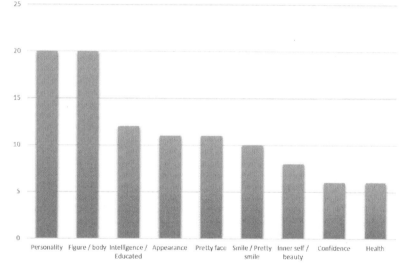

No matter how we personally rank these ingredients in order of importance, finding a good balance across all four areas is essential. The following four chapters will provide clear directions on how to get you there. Some of the advice and best practices may appear quite sound, even commonsense. You may also discover new ideas that will profoundly change your perspective on how you approach life. Follow the advice you'll find there, and listen to the pearls you met earlier.

You may not master all four of these qualities right away, but they're now within reach. Luckily, you've accomplished a major step by reading this book—you're now much closer to realizing how beautiful you REALLY are.

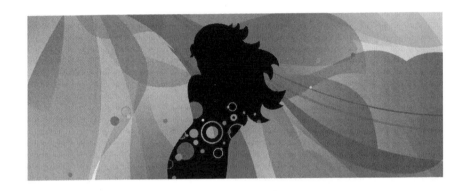

*"Although beauty may be
in the eye of the beholder,
the feeling of being beautiful
exists solely in the mind of the beheld."*

**- Martha Beck,
American sociologist and therapist**

CHAPTER FOUR

FEELING GOOD—
NOT JUST LOOKING GOOD

Born in Richland, Washington, a mile from the Hanford nuclear site, Hope Solo was conceived during one of her mother's conjugal visits to Walla Walla State Penitentiary. This self-proclaimed "country girl" is no stranger to adversity. Solo's parents divorced when she was only six and her father, an Italian-American Vietnam War veteran, was in and out of prison throughout her childhood.

The young Hope Solo didn't let these challenges stop her from pursuing her dreams—she became one of the most famous women's soccer players and the best goalkeeper in the world. Coached by her father from the age of five, Solo began her soccer career as a forward at high school in Richland, leading her team to the state championships and three consecutive league titles. She realized that soccer was her ticket to a college education, as she "knew my family couldn't afford to send me to college." On the University of Washington's soccer team, she became the best goalie in Pac-10 history, setting numerous records.

Solo's track record speaks for itself. She helped her team win gold at the 2008 Summer Olympics in Beijing, just nine months after a major surgery. She was starting goalkeeper for the U.S. in the 2007 and 2011 FIFA Women's World Cup. Always quick on her feet, she even appeared on the 13th season of *Dancing with the Stars* in 2011, with dancing partner Maksim Chmerkovskiy. Solo has been featured on countless cover magazines, from *Vogue* to *Fitness*. When asked about her semi-nude appearance in The Body Issue of *ESPN The Magazine* in 2011, she said,

I'm an athlete—that's all I am. If a sex symbol is now a top female athlete, I think that's pretty amazing and it shows how far our country has come from the stick-thin models, from what you see in most magazines.

Solo's personality, direct style and charisma propelled her to celebrity status among women. Other than Serena Williams, she has been Googled more than any other female athlete in the world. She proved that endurance is a quality needed not just on the field, but in life too. The traits shaped by her childhood—hard work, resilience and toughness—proved to be amazing assets.

Solo understands better than anyone that being fully equipped to pursue your dreams requires eating a balanced diet, exercising regularly, getting adequate sleep and taking care of your skin. In the Nike Women "Make Yourself" campaign, Solo focuses on combining endurance, cardio and strength in her exercise routine. A celebrity spokesperson for the Simple Skincare brand, she knows how hard it is to maintain healthy skin, especially with an active lifestyle. Solo has become a role model to many, making it clear how exercise and healthy lifestyles enhance girls' and women's lives.

Perhaps the most common misconception among women today is that getting to the right size or body shape is the key to being— or simply feeling—beautiful. Women value being physically healthy and having a balanced lifestyle—sleeping, eating and exercising— but struggle to make it a daily routine. According to a study by the American Psychological Association:

- Although 75 percent of women believe sleep is important, only 33 percent report getting enough of it
- Although 64 percent of women believe eating healthy is important, only 36 percent actually do it
- Although 54 percent of women believe being physically active is important, only 29 percent actually are.

Every day, the gap between what we know and what we actually *do* seems to widen—and that just adds to our stress levels.

It's a constant challenge to stay focused on health rather than just looks when you're bombarded by messages that place a premium on obtaining the "perfect body" no matter what. No one knows this better than Cameron Russell, a Victoria's Secret favorite who has appeared in multiple international editions of *Vogue* and ads for brands like Ralph Lauren and Benetton. In her TED Talk "Looks Aren't Everything, Believe Me I Am a Model," Russell challenges what it means to have the body we are "biologically programmed to admire." She warns, "You just need to meet a group of models, because they have the thinnest thighs and the shiniest hair and the coolest clothes, and they're the most physically insecure women probably on the planet." Russell is right: looks aren't everything. But a strong, healthy body is essential to pursuing our goals in life.

Where should we look for answers?

No one's to blame for feeling confused about our endless quest for health and beauty. Virtually thousands of books exist to help women of all ages build their ideal body, or get in the best shape of their lives. Hundreds of so-called miracle diets promise to help you drop a size or two . . . and to reenergize you in the process. You've heard it all, and more. Countless glamour and fashion magazines, articles, books, infomercials and a multitude of online resources offer endless advice on the three Fs assumed to be women's best friends: food, fitness and fashion. The amount of resources and contradictory advice might just make your head spin.

> *"The secret to being healthy is to avoid depriving yourself. Don't starve yourself or only eat veggies. I eat six times a day to stay energized. By the way, peanut M&Ms are okay as long as you eat those in moderation. Balance and a healthy lifestyle are key ingredients."*
>
> *- Kristen Dalton*

Most recommendations made by self-proclaimed health and food experts are common sense. But new concepts and ideas in fitness and nutrition (gluten-free, low-carb, no sugar, H2O diets, detoxes) make headlines every day, insisting that we had it all wrong all along. Still unclear about what advice to follow? You're not alone.

> *"The secret of a strong, healthy body is eating well. I juice every morning fresh organic vegetables and fruits, from green apples, carrots, ginger, kale and romaine salad. Don't focus on what you can't eat but instead on the abundance of great food available to you."*
> *- Susie Castillo*

We are all different. We are each unique.

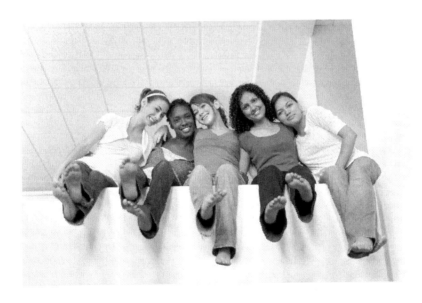

We all want to be healthy and energized, and to feel great in our bodies. We're conditioned to believe that by following the same meal plan, the same fitness program and the same sleeping schedule, we should all arrive at the same outcome. It's important, though, to remember that everyone's different. Genetics greatly influence bone structure, frame size, shape, height and weight. The DNA lottery has gifted each of us with different assets. We each have a different genetic inheritance, ethnic and cultural traits—and therefore we respond differently to eating and exercising. The same exact amount of food, sleep and exercise will produce very different results for two different people. The answer lies in each and every one of us. Sadly, there is no silver-bullet answer to the question, "what is the secret to a healthy body?" Yet struggles over our looks can drain our overall outlook and enjoyment of life—not to mention our productivity.

How do we avoid falling into that trap? We must first avoid the common mistake of comparing our body to others, whether they are close friends, supermodels or perfect strangers in the street. Comparing ourselves to others only leads to low self-esteem, lack of confidence, jealousy and even resentment. There's always someone out there with a fitter body and a faster metabolism.

> *"Go all in. Never stop. Push yourself to the limits. Working out with friends helps. Allow your routine to change the way you live your life. Drinks lots and lots of water. Practice relaxation regularly. Have a healthy diet. And remember that sleep is critical."*
>
> *- Heidi Forrest*

How we look and feel is the result of complex circumstances that arise from a combination of long-standing biological, behavioral, psychological, interpersonal and social factors. In other words, there's much more than meets the eye. For most people, it's not as simple as saying, "I want to look my best" and being disciplined about eating, sleeping, exercising and skincare. How we look is an intimate part of who we are, or who we want to become. We must focus our efforts and energy on being the best version of ourselves—and feel great about it.

How do we each determine "the right body" for us? The ideal body is the one that lets us feel strong and energetic. It lets us lead a healthy, active life. Your body is a complex, custom-made vehicle that moves you through everyday life. It must be well attended to and carefully nurtured. It may not always feel like it's perfect—but it's probably much stronger and healthier than you think. It's very tempting to take shortcuts like fad diets and reinvent ourselves to conform to societal standards. Too many women use cosmetic surgery to buy their way to the body of their dreams. Instead, we must learn to appreciate and emphasize what's unique and special in each of us. Sometimes, what we don't like about our appearance turns out to be what others find most charming and truly special about us. Let's learn to embrace and cultivate our physical differences.

> *"If you feel the best, you look your best. It's that simple."*
>
> *- Heidi Forrest*

Key ingredients for a strong, healthy body

Eating right, exercising regularly, sleeping enough and adequate skincare contribute not just to your physical and emotional health, but to your overall wellbeing. You don't have to be a rocket scientist from NASA to know that. Yet the simple things can be the hardest to put into practice. We're full of good intentions at the beginning of the year: our New Year's resolutions often feature promises about diet, exercise and sleep. We know it's the right thing to do—we know we will live longer and better lives if we do. Yet we quickly fall back into life routines and daily temptations. We get busy. We get distracted. And we forget! We make up hundreds of excuses (yes, I've been there too). We postpone our resolutions one more day, one more week, even one more year.

> *"Because I barely stand five feet tall, I started limiting myself because of my height. Then I realized that I can do all things with God. The only person who is limiting me is myself. I have the wisdom, talent, creativity to be excellent in whatever I set my mind to."*
>
> *- Maureen Francisco*

Here's the bad news: we don't have the luxury to wait that long. Stop making excuses. Although you can't change your genetics, you can always change your health and your habits. Focus on what you *can* change and make it happen. It's vital to treat your body with respect each and every day: consider it your most valuable asset and your number-one priority. It's also your most fragile asset. Of course, your own personal health and medical conditions, lifestyle and professional environment determine what your own body needs. Whether you're moderately active or a competitive athlete, whether you want to gain strength or increase muscle size, whether you want to maintain or improve your eating habits, all determine how to nourish and condition your body.

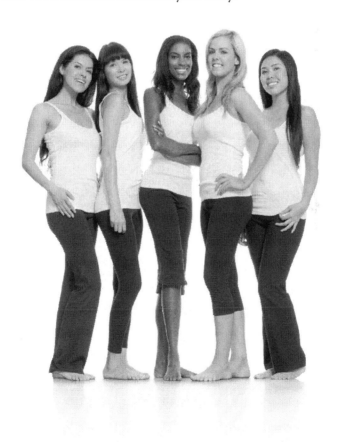

It's no surprise that highly successful women have developed a positive, sustainable balance of eating, exercise and healthy activities. Those elements support self-esteem, confidence, a sense of competence and control. We have a strong, healthy relationship with our body when we understand and appreciate our natural body's characteristics, feel comfortable in it, and recognize that our appearance has little to do with our character or value.

When we nourish our body, we have the stamina and energy to think, concentrate, interact with others, engage in sports or hobbies and wake up energized. Here are the ingredients for success as shown in the "Body Journey Wheel of Success" below:

- **FUEL:** Eating smarter for healthier living
- **BURN:** Getting fit for life
- **REST:** Building healthy sleep habits
- **REPAIR:** Nurturing skin for a radiant look

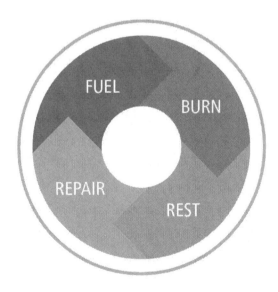

Figure: Body Journey Wheel of Success

FUEL

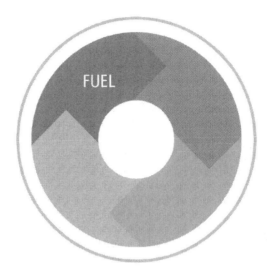

A healthy lifestyle begins with a balance of nutritious meals and regular physical activity. Think of food as the fuel your body needs to operate. To keep running efficiently, your car needs quality fuel and plenty of fluids. So does your body. Your body needs water, vitamins and nutrient-rich foods from a variety of food groups to release the energy it needs to function. French playwright and actor Jean-Baptiste Poquelin (1622–1673), known by his stage name Molière, wisely reminded us that "One should eat to live, not live to eat." Unfortunately, most Americans are overfed and yet craving food more than ever: we get high calories and low nutrition. The quality of fuel you put in your body directly impacts your performance. Carla Sanchez of Performance Ready says it best: "Eat naturally lean, powerfully green and fatty clean!" Low-quality food will yield low-quality output: garbage in, garbage out. Overcooked, over-processed and chemically manipulated foods that come in a box or a can have little-to-no nutritional value.

> "A common mistake people make is eating excessive processed food. Remember that the easier it is to digest what you eat, the healthier you will be."
>
> - Susie Castillo

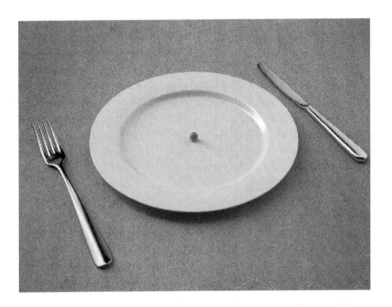

If you eat smart, you don't need to be on a diet. Actually, dieting is for the most part a physiologically flawed concept that produces negative effects. If you've tried diets and exercise programs with less-than-satisfying results, you've learned what so many women know: though it's a multi-billion dollar industry, dieting simply doesn't work for most people to produce sustainable, long-term results. Studies have shown that 90-95 percent of dieters gain back the weight they lose—sometimes they gain even more. Every time we lose weight by dieting, our body responds by trying to protect us from the possible effects of "starvation," so it slows down our metabolism and adds extra body fat as insurance. We may lose 5 or 10 pounds on a diet, but we're likely to gain back more.

In her popular TED Talk, Sandra Aamodt makes it clear "Why dieting doesn't usually work." She explains that:

Several long-term studies have shown that girls who diet in their early teenage years are three times more likely to become overweight five years later, even if they started at a normal weight.

Aamodt adds (again based on various studies) that:

Diets don't have very much reliability. Five years after a diet, most people have regained the weight or have gained even more. If you think about this, the typical outcome of dieting is that you're more likely to gain weight in the long run than to lose it.

Many dieters feel that they don't lose weight even when they eat less. While "quantity" does matter, many still over-consume calories, sugar and artificial ingredients by choosing the wrong foods. Eating the *right* foods is essential—yet so many of us don't know what those right foods are, due to conflicting messages we receive from the news, food industry lobbies and health professionals. Many women experience damaging emotions, attitudes and behaviors surrounding weight and food; some suffer from eating disorders such as anorexia and bulimia.

> "*I am always most productive when I rest. Don't stress out. Take the time to take care of yourself. Health is #1 for me. Get enough sleep, eat the right food. You don't need to be a size 2 but stay healthy*"
>
> *- Marika Siewert*

Don't judge your health or your worth by a number on the scale. Should you pay attention to food and calories? Of course: we all need to be aware of our food intake, especially when it comes to carbs and calorie-dense foods. But occasional wine, bread, chocolate and cheese won't hurt you.

In her book *French Women Don't Get Fat,* author Mireille Guiliano explains this "French paradox": how French women stay slim and healthy even though they enjoy bread and pastry, wine, regular three-course meals and chocolate. Few people know about the fat-burning benefits associated with antioxidant-rich concentrated (a minimum of 70% cacao) dark chocolate. Yes: a moderate amount of chocolate can do you good. (But don't attempt a French diet that includes regular chocolate croissants and *eclairs au chocolat-it* won't turn out so well!) The reality is that French people also drink a lot of water: Evian, Perrier, Badoit, Contrex and Volvic are familiar names on French kitchen tables. They enjoy fresh local products. They eat vegetables and fruits in reasonable quantities. They eat slowly, over extended lunches or dinners, and in much smaller quantities.

> *"Feeling beautiful is important to me, as it is for most women. We want to feel good, be desired and more importantly, we want to feel valued. Beauty is an asset but it can't be the only thing you focus on. You simply want to be the best version of you, love yourself and surround yourself with people who love your beauty, on the inside and out."*
>
> *- Kristen Dalton*

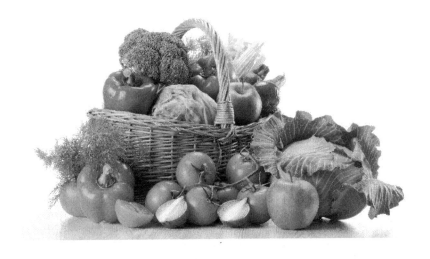

Only use top-quality ingredients, free from hormones, antibiotics and preservatives. Healthier buying habits and the rapid growth of organic brands is a sign that consumers are getting wiser about their food intake. They're also more vocal and more influential as they demand healthier ingredients from food manufacturers.

> *"Get your proteins through natural resources and stay away from processed food."*
>
> *- Brittany Dawn Brannon*

This isn't a food book, so I won't be sharing exotic recipes or providing Nutrition 101 lessons. There are thousands of books on the subject—unfortunately, many of them lack scientific data to support their claims. A search on Amazon.com for "food" revealed approximately 280,000 results. If you search for "diet" you'll see over 95,000 titles—for every three books on food, you'll find one on diet. If you read one book per week, it would take you over 1,800 years to read the existing inventory of diet books on Amazon.com—and they publish more every day. So pace yourself, and choose carefully!

If you plan to read any book about nutrition, I'd suggest the following quality reads and valuable resources:

- *In Defense of Food, Food Rules* and *The Omnivore's Dilemma* by Michael Pollan
- *Power Eating* (fourth edition) and *The Good Mood Diet* by Dr. Susan Kleiner
- *Disease Proof: The Remarkable Truth about What Makes Us Well* by Dr. David Katz
- *Food Politics* and *What to Eat* by Dr. Marion Nestle.

In the end, health is in your hands. Here are some things to consider for the healthiest way to FUEL your body:

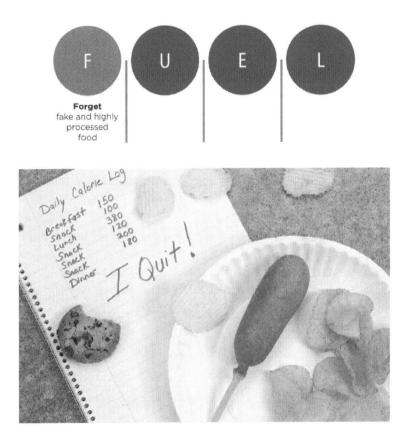

F **U** **E** **L**

Forget
fake and highly
processed
food

1.   **F**orget fake and highly processed foods. Stay away from foods that
     contain artificial colors, flavors or sweeteners. Avoid excessive addi-
     tives, food coloring and sugar. Processed food has become a multi-
     billion dollar industry that makes our lives easier but our health
     poorer. Sadly, it's everywhere around us, conveniently within reach
     and without much preparation needed. Food additives such as artifi-
     cial sweeteners, high-fructose corn syrup (HFCS), hydrogenated oils
     and MSG can lead to food addiction, obesity, and increased risk for
     chronic disease. MSG (monosodium glutamate), an addictive food
     additive, is added to 80 percent of all flavored foods. It's also used to
     fatten up mice for scientific study. If you want to achieve your ideal
     body weight and health, avoid fast foods and other known junk foods
     as well as these food additives at all costs.

"Drink a lot of water and make sure to have a nutritious, well-rounded diet. I eat all kinds of food but no meat. I stay away from eating too much processed food."

- Melanie Kannokada

Are we addicted to additives? Sweeteners (both artificial and sugar-derived) top the list of addictive additives and are very unhealthy for the body. Aspartame, sold under the brand names NutraSweet and Equal, is often combined with caffeine in diet cola; this creates a very addictive combination that gives us a slight buzz, yet offers no nutritional value. You also want to limit your sodium intake—consider alternatives like citrus or fresh herbs for flavor. The more real foods from nature you eat, the less packaged and processed foods you'll consume and the more energy you'll have.

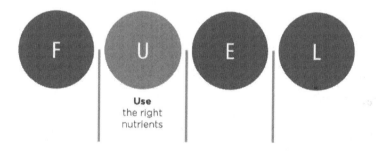

Use the right nutrients

2. Use the right nutrients. Eat whole fruits and vegetables (preferably organic or fresh local produce) along with nuts and seeds. It's easy to go overboard with fruits, as we tend to favor those over vegetables. Remember, though, that fruits have about three times the average calorie count of vegetables; most people should not exceed three servings per day to maintain a reasonable sugar intake and not gain weight. Consider getting a juicer (or better, a blender like Vitamix, Blendtec or KitchenAid) to absorb even more antioxidants and nutrients—it's a great way to start the day with endless tasty recipes. For a healthy meal, choose seafood, lean meats and poultry whenever possible. Eat whole-grain products like whole wheat, brown rice and quinoa.

According to the USDA's new food-guidance system (you can find it at choosemyplate.gov), 50% of our diet should come from fruits and vegetables, and a more moderate 30% from grains. Some advocate reducing grains down to 15% and increasing protein intake from 20% to at least 35%, citing benefits from added protein including better blood sugar control, a decrease in body fat and an increase in calorie-burning lean muscle. If you stay within these USDA general guidelines, you'll set yourself up for healthy eating habits.

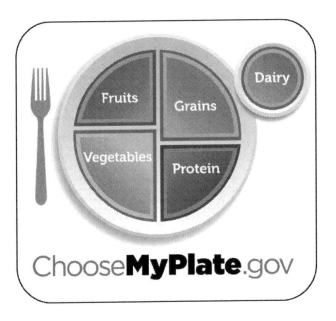

Some experts believe the USDA guidelines to be flawed, including Cassandra Forsythe, the author of two popular, nationally publicized books for women: *The New Rules of Lifting for Women* and *Women's Health Perfect Body Diet*. Forsythe holds a PhD in Exercise Science and Nutrition and is a registered dietitian. She's known for her expertise in low-carb diets, nutrition for fat loss, and all aspects of women's health; she's been featured in major magazines such as *Oxygen* and *Women's Health*. Forsythe says that the USDA guidance:

doesn't encourage people to choose unprocessed foods over whole items, because it still suggests that we eat frozen meals (that we probably microwave in a plastic container); and doesn't address our over-consumption of sugar in snacks, desserts, and hidden in common foods like breads and salad dressings.

Instead, Forsythe says we should choose natural, unprocessed proteins from animal or vegetable sources, and dairy that's not loaded with sugar. She recommends filling half your plate with fresh or cooked vegetables, a quarter with fresh fruit, whole grains (never processed), and the rest with natural fats like olive oil, nuts, or meat and fish oils.

Julianne Hough, an American actress, country music singer and professional ballroom dancer, is also a two-time professional champion of ABC's *Dancing with the Stars*. She's known to follow a strict diet and exercise regime that has contributed to her healthy looks and lifestyle. She's also a fan of superfoods, saying, "I've incorporated superfoods into my diet to keep me healthy, from the inside out. In addition to all the dancing I'm doing, I want to make sure that what goes into my body is nutritious as well."

Use nutrients that best support your lifestyle. If you're active, get enough fluid, carbs and a protein-heavy snack after exercising. Sports nutritionists suggest that taking these three elements immediately after an hour-long workout might contribute to better recovery and refueling of the body.

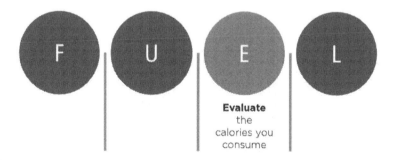

Evaluate
the
calories you
consume

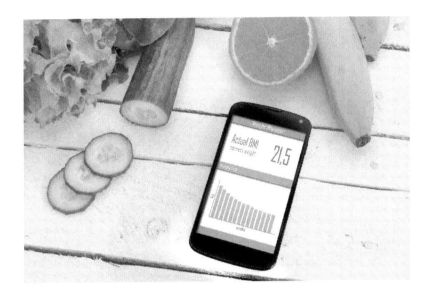

3. Evaluate the calories you consume. Keep track of the calories, sugar and fat you eat to help you maintain your weight or reach whatever goal you've set. There are many great Smartphone apps like "Lose It!," an easy-to-use program that helps you stay within your calorie budget. It's always healthiest to focus on preventing weight gain instead of encouraging weight loss. You can enjoy vibrant health, abundant energy, and achieve your ideal body weight without dieting.

Indian-born American cookbook author, actress, model and television host Padma Lakshmi knows a thing or two about eating well. She's been the host of Bravo's reality TV show *Top Chef* since 2006. Once a model for top designers such as Ralph Lauren and Giorgio Armani, she also wrote cookbooks such as the award-winning *Easy Exotic,* a compilation of international recipes. In *Fitness Magazine,* Lakshmi described her balanced exercising and eating program: "I follow a clean diet: no meats, no sweets, no alcohol, no cheese, no fried food, and no wheat. And I work out five days a week, boxing three days, lifting weights the other two." Brought up as a vegetarian, Lakshmi added: "I love food way too much to starve myself just to look good. I will put in the work at the gym so I can enjoy what I eat." She keeps an eye on her calorie consumption, but refuses to suffer.

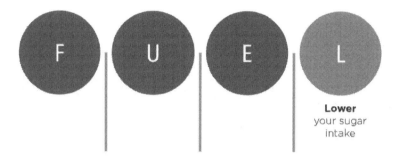

Lower
your sugar
intake

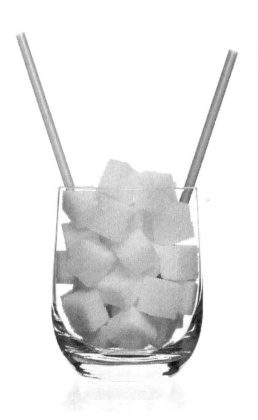

4. Lower your sugar intake. We tend to consume too much fructose, primarily in the form of high-fructose corn syrup. It's our largest source of calories—what's more, it's addictive. Sugar causes a

beta-endorphin rush in your brain, with morphine-like physiological effects. When we're feeling down or stressed out, we gravitate towards "comfort foods" that lift our mood. As with any drug, our body becomes dependent, requiring more sugar over time to get the same result. When we consume too much sugar, our pancreas has to secrete large amounts of insulin to bring our blood sugar level down again. That sugar is then turned into fat so it can be stored.

> *"Beauty is important to me. It's how I take care of myself internally - spiritually, emotionally, and psychologically - and externally - physically. I'm responsible for taking care of the mind/body that God gave me for the rest of my life."*
>
> *- Maureen Francisco*

Yet much of that fructose is hidden in all types of processed foods and beverages (everyday products like bread, cereal, salad dressing and pasta sauce), so it's hard to avoid. Control your sugar intake so it doesn't become harmful. And watch out for fruit juices and smoothies: they may sound healthy, but most are loaded with sugar.

The FUEL principle is actually quite simple. You can pursue health naturally by gradually replacing processed "faux-food" with organic, nutrient-dense real foods, and by making other lifestyle changes like getting regular exercise and reducing daily stress. And remember: eating well is a permanent lifestyle change.

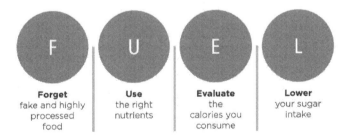

F
Forget
fake and highly processed food

U
Use
the right nutrients

E
Evaluate
the calories you consume

L
Lower
your sugar intake

Apply the following recommendations by one of the country's top nutritionists and you'll be well on your way to successfully FUEL your body.

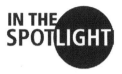

Top Five Recommendations by Expert Nutritionist Susan M. Kleiner, PhD, RD, FACN, CNS, FISSN:

1. **Feed your body, fuel your mind.** Follow the power-eating paradigm: EAT MORE-GAIN ENERGY-TRAIN HARDER-BUILD MUSCLE-BURN FAT FOR GOOD!

2. **Fully fuel your training, then eat mindfully the rest of the day.** No need for counting grams or calories, or restricting. Let hunger and satisfaction be your guides.

3. **Think about what you NEED to eat, not what you can't eat next.** Eat an omnivorous diet, abundant in plant foods grown close to home and minimally processed.

4. **Drink at least 5-6 cups of pure water every day, and at least 9-11 cups of total fluids.** Drink more to hydrate around exercise, travel, illness, hot climate or pregnancy/lactation.

5. **Put your food to work for you:** Combine carbohydrates, protein and high-performance fat-rich foods together at every meal and snack. This will feed your muscles and fuel your brain for mind-body energy, elevated mood, clear thinking and enhanced rest.

BURN

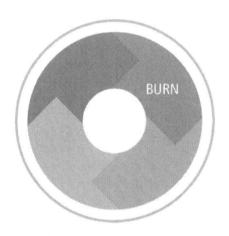

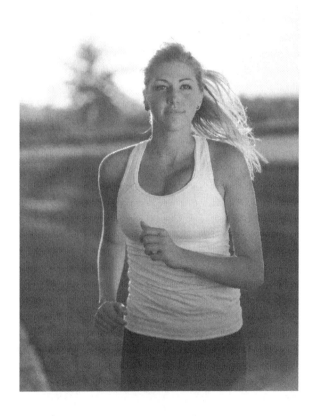

Choosing which foods to eat is important, but it's not the whole picture. Modern life has become so convenient that we have fewer chances to be physically active. Instead of walking, we ride in cars. Instead of running to the mall, we shop online. Most of us sit in an office chair for more than six hours a day. If we do, our risk of heart disease increases by up to 64 percent, and we shave off seven years of quality life. So in our ultra-convenient culture, regular and moderate physical activity—30 to 60 minutes every day—has health benefits that are hard to ignore. There's a reason why you've heard "exercise is good for you" ever since you were a child: it was true then, and now it's even more critical to your health.

> *"If you exercise, don't go crazy on the first week or you will plateau quickly. Tone your body over time"*
>
> *- Connor Boss*

Exercise is good for you on many levels. It metabolizes your stress hormones, boosts energy and endurance, reduces hunger, improves muscle strength, helps you sleep better and longer, and contributes to your overall wellbeing. It also helps prevent a wide range of serious health problems: high blood pressure, cholesterol and type 2 diabetes, to name a few. Women are particularly prone to osteoporosis or weakened bones as they age; exercise helps keep your bones strong and healthy. It also helps reduce the risk of depression—it improves your mood by stimulating brain chemicals and helping you relax after a long day. For some, exercise helps prevent excess weight gain and promotes weight loss. Others use it to tone their thighs, develop six-pack abs or build better muscle definition on their arms, legs or glutes.

Simple, everyday activities contribute to a healthy level of exercise. Having an exercise routine helps a lot, whether you enjoy running, jumping, biking, dancing, walking or anything in between. The options are endless, and exploring them can be fun—hot yoga, anyone? Equipped with climate-controlled facilities, friendly staff and cutting-edge technology, gyms can be a perfect solution, especially in winter. But plenty of healthy adventures await those who'd rather get their exercise outdoors.

"Doing cardio every single day made me gain weight. Instead, I recommend doing weights 3 to 4 times a week and following a well-balanced cardio-to-weight training program"
- Brittany Dawn Brannon

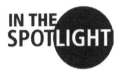

IN THE SPOTLIGHT

The Truth about Exercise

Like most people, you may rush to the treadmill after sitting at your desk the whole day. But can three minutes of exercise a week help make you fit? British journalist and physician Michael Mosley takes us on a journey to uncover the truth about exercise in a PBS documentary.

Mosley reveals the latest scientific discoveries about how bodies respond to a workout, and why different people respond differently. Using himself as a guinea pig, he shares surprising new research which suggests many of us could benefit from just three minutes of intense training (such as high-intensity cycling) a week. Benefits were measured based on insulin sensitivity (how well insulin removes sugar from the blood and controls fat) and aerobic fitness (how good your heart and lungs are at getting oxygen into your body).

Mosley's key finding: it's better to move actively throughout the day, with activities like walking, than to sit still an entire day and hit the gym in the evening.

Here are some easy-to-follow ways to build exercising into your busy everyday life. Just remember to BURN!

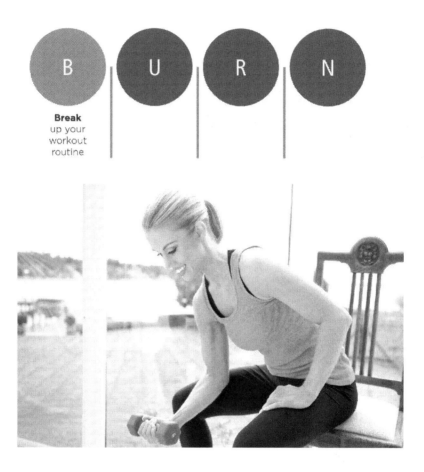

Break
up your
workout
routine

1. **B**reak up your workout routine. Alternate your exercise routine to work on your cardio and muscle tone—you need both. Cardio-strengthening activities like running or bicycling build strong heart muscle and endurance. Muscle-strengthening activities like push-ups, sit-ups and weightlifting make your muscles stronger. It's important to work all the different parts of your body: your legs, hips, back, chest, stomach, shoulders and arms. Bone-strengthening activities like jumping promote bone growth and strength. Balance and stretching activities like dance and yoga enhance physical stability and flexibility, reducing your risk of injury. Trying different kinds of exercise on alternate days helps keep things interesting and lessens the chance

of getting hurt. Every little bit adds up, and doing *something* is a lot better than doing nothing.

> "Work out hard but give your body enough time to rest. Eat something every 3 to 4 hours. Make sure to get enough high protein and low carb nutrition. Vegetables and fruits are always a must."
>
> - Connor Boss

Danica Patrick is an auto-racing driver, model and advertising spokeswoman—she knows how to live life in the fast lane. Although auto racing is considered more of a mental game, physical strength and endurance are essential for hours of competitive racing around a NASCAR track. She lifts weights three days a week to stay strong, alternating between upper and lower body. In an interview in *Fitness Magazine,* she revealed,

> My routine includes a lot of functional training, like squats and lunges with an upper body move, for core stabilization. Cardio is also important, and it feels good to work my lungs and breathe deep.

Patrick, whose image has graced the cover of many magazines including the *Sports Illustrated* swimsuit issue, knows to keep her body in shape by breaking up her workout routine. She isn't afraid to take on the boys of NASCAR: she's considered the most successful woman in the history of American open-wheel racing.

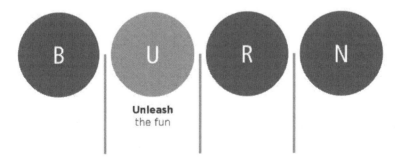

Unleash
the fun

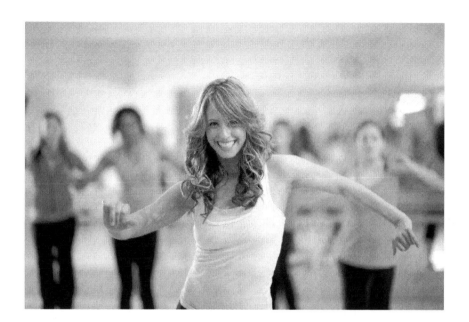

2. **U**nleash the fun. Have you ever dragged your feet to the gym? Have you ever had to push yourself to go exercise? You're not alone—but there are ways to make it more enjoyable. Explore different forms of exercise: share your workout with close friends and consider team activities to keep it exciting. More importantly, have fun doing it! It's so easy to get bored or simply burn out when it becomes a constant military-style drill. To be ready any time, keep comfortable clothes, a pair of walking or running shoes, and sports equipment in the car and at the office. Be open when others ask you to join them. Try something you haven't before. Look for ways to combine your workouts with fun, and you'll never have to exercise again. What a concept, isn't it? Apply yourself, but don't take yourself too seriously!

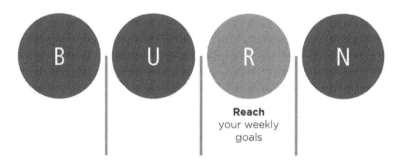

Reach
your weekly
goals

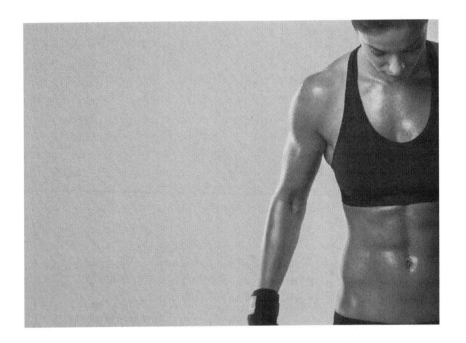

3. **R**each your weekly goals. Set aside 30-60 minutes each day for exercise; five or more hours of activity each week provide even more health benefits. Combine high- and low-impact activities to reduce strain on your knees and joints. You can choose moderate (dancing or brisk walking) or vigorous activities (swimming or running), or mix it up each week based on your personal goals and preferences.

Fitting exercise into your daily routine can be easy. Choose activities you enjoy and that you can do regularly. Check resources like *Shape* or *Fitness Magazine* for workouts—abs, shoulders, arms, back, butt, thighs, legs and more. Get a membership at a local gym—you'll no longer have excuses when it's cold or dark. Most gyms have a wide range of equipment for both cardio and strengthening activities.

> *"Always give a first great impression. Taking good care of your body is essential. Hold your head high and more importantly, always feel confident about how you look."*
>
> - Susie Castillo

Everything is easier when you set goals. Ask Lindsey Vonn. A talented alpine ski racer on the U.S. Ski Team, she has won four World Cup championships and the gold medal in downhill at the 2010 Winter Olympics. Considered the most successful American woman ski racer in history, Vonn's remarkable dedication despite her numerous injuries led to endorsement deals with marquee brands like Oakley, Red Bull, Rolex and Under Armour. She caused a stir when she swapped her skis for a bikini, appearing in the 2010 *Sports Illustrated* swimsuit edition along with other Winter Olympians.

Vonn's recipe for success is a commitment to practice and training. She skis often to perfect her technical skills and speed, but incorporates a diverse workout when she's indoors—endurance cycling, tight-rope walking and reaction training. "I do everything I can to get in shape," she admitted to *Fitness Magazine*. And it shows. Vonn's a great example of someone who doesn't just look great but *feels* great too. She uses her body to bring women's skiing to a new level of performance by setting specific weekly goals and working hard to meet them.

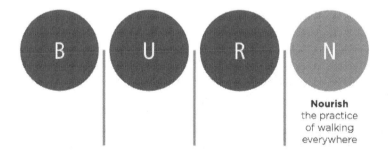

Nourish
the practice
of walking
everywhere

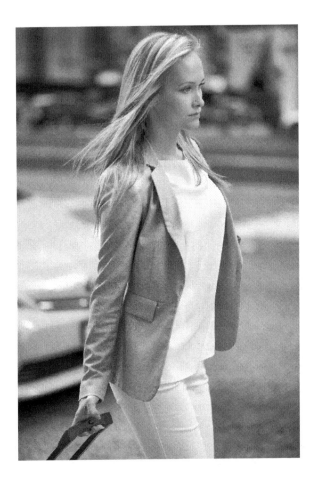

4. **N**ourish the practice of walking everywhere. In her TED Talk "Got a Meeting? Take a Walk," Nilofer Merchant explains, nowadays people are sitting 9.3 hours a day, which is more than we're sleeping, at 7.7 hours. Sitting is so incredibly prevalent, we don't even question how much we're doing it, and because everyone else is doing it, it doesn't even occur to us that it's not okay. In that way, sitting has become the smoking of our generation.

To address this problem, Merchant suggests that we get moving during our social interactions. Consider conducting your next meeting on a walk. Walk to work, to the subway, to the grocery store. Simply walking the dog for 10 minutes before and after work, or adding a 10-minute walk at lunchtime, can add to your weekly goal. Make it fun too. Consider apps like "The Walk," a fitness tracker and game combined. It's more than just a great pedometer/step counter—it's a way to turn walking into a rip-roaring adventure that spices up step-tracking with danger and intrigue across 65 episodes, 800 minutes of audio and hundreds of miles. When you're playing "The Walk," every step counts; the app helps you walk more, every single day. Save the world and start walking everywhere.

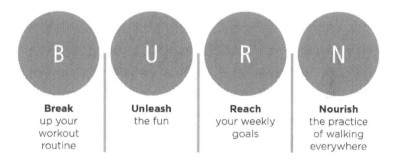

Break
up your
workout
routine

Unleash
the fun

Reach
your weekly
goals

Nourish
the practice
of walking
everywhere

Adopt the following recommendations by a top fitness expert and you'll have a stronger body before you know it.

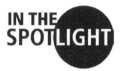

IN THE
SPOTLIGHT

Top Five Recommendations by Fitness Expert Linda Melone, CSCS:

1. **Move as much as you can.** Structured exercise isn't always possible, so take advantage of any opportunities to move: Conduct walking meetings. Park far from your office building and walk briskly to the front door. Take the stairs instead of the elevator. Get up from your desk to talk on the phone. It all adds up to calories burned and better health overall.

2. **Find a social aspect to your workouts.** Even if you're an introvert like me, finding other people who share your love of a particular class, sport or activity keeps you going on days you'd rather skip it. A workout partner can also help hold you accountable. But simply being around others who expect you to show up can be highly motivating.

3. **Be realistic.** Many people quit three to six months after starting a workout program because they set their sights too high. Establish goals you can achieve. Don't expect to lose 10 pounds in a week or fit into a pant size you haven't seen since your 20s. Make goals you can control, such as walking X times a week versus losing X number of pounds, which can be unpredictable. Results will happen if you stick to it.

4. **Be consistent.** Avoid being a weekend warrior or someone who works out only to lose weight. See exercise and activity as life-long ventures to help you function better in everything you do. Do something every day, even if it's a 10-minute walk or a set of quick push-ups and squats during your lunch break.

5. **Add variety.** Doing a monotonous treadmill workout every day can quickly put the kibosh on the best of intentions. Find a few options you enjoy. If you walk, check out new walking paths, join a walking club once or twice a week, or find a walking partner. If you also enjoy swimming, make that a second option. If you can't change your location, add new music, buy a new workout outfit or try a different program. Find ways to keep your head in the game for the rest of your life.\

REST

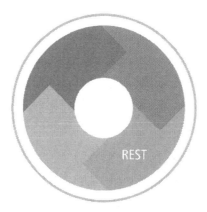

It's a well-known challenge. We're all desperately sleep-deprived in today's 24-hour, "always-on" society. The National Sleep Foundation conducted a sleep survey from 1999-2004. Here's what they found: 40 million Americans suffer from over 70 different sleep disorders (from apnea to restless legs syndrome); 60% of adults have sleep problems a few times a week. Most people sleep less than six hours a night. Women in particular face so many personal and professional demands that few get enough sleep.

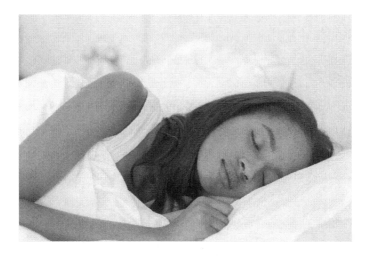

We all know well that sleep is important—but we may not know just *how* important. Humans have an internal clock that mirrors nature's cycles of day and night. Quality sleep is essential to physical and emotional wellbeing, and to healthy body and brain function. It helps repair heart and blood vessels, cells and tissue. Deep sleep is a great way to neutralize stress hormones. Stress increases fluid retention—you can gain up to two pounds in body fluids just from one night of stress-induced sleeplessness! Restful sleep helps recharge our batteries and decrease fatigue.

Chronic lack of sleep—or poor quality sleep—increases your risk of health issues such as diabetes, heart problems, hypertension, weight gain and obesity, and psychiatric conditions like depression and substance abuse. It leads to moodiness, impatience, an inability to concentrate, and negatively impacts performance, creativity, problem solving and decision-making. If you want to protect your brain and body from toxicity, wear and potential damage, you need to get enough rest.

> *"Someone may be exceptionally physically beautiful but could be ugly on the inside. How you present yourself totally matters, not only how you look. This is essential to you getting the things you want and need in life. "*
>
> - Heidi Forrest

At the University of Rochester Medical Center, researchers discovered that it's during sleep that the brain clears out potentially harmful waste that builds up during the day. Because this process is so energy intensive, the brain can't do this during the day while it's in high-activity mode and preoccupied with performing everyday tasks.

In a thought-provoking TED Talk, Arianna Huffington jokingly invites women to "sleep your way to the top." She proposes "a small idea that can awaken much bigger ones: the power of a good night's sleep." Instead of bragging about sleep deficits, she urges us to shut our eyes and see the big picture: "We can sleep our way to increased productivity and happiness—and smarter decision-making."

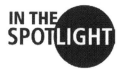

IN THE SPOTLIGHT

Why We Need Sleep

In his TED Talk, "Why Do We Sleep?" circadian neuroscientist Russell Foster explains that "if you're an average sort of person, 36 percent of your life will be spent asleep, which means that if you live to 90, then 32 years will have been spent entirely asleep."

Foster studies the sleep cycles of the brain. He argues that—despite what many of us think—sleep is not a waste of time. "Actually," he says, "sleep is an incredibly important part of our biology." In his eye-opening talk, Foster explains that we are likely sleep-deprived if: we need an alarm clock to get us out of bed in the morning, we take a long time to get up, we need lots of stimulants, we're grumpy or irritable, or we're told by our colleagues or friends that we're looking tired and irritable.

Foster also speaks to the connection between sleep loss and weight gain. If we sleep five hours or less every night, we have a 50-percent chance of being obese. Why? Sleep loss seems to cause a release of the hormone ghrelin, the hunger hormone. The brain hears, "I need carbo-hydrates"—and it seeks out carbs, particularly sugars. As if we needed another reason to sleep, this link between sleeplessness and a predisposition for weight gain can't be ignored.

Here are the most important ways to get the REST you need:

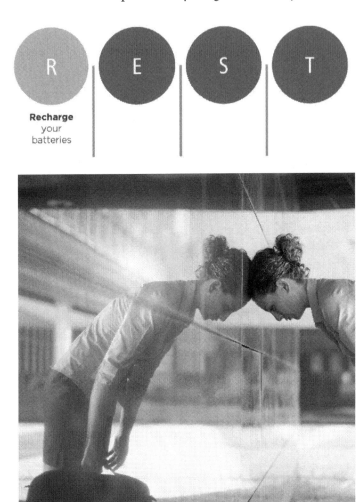

1. **R**echarge your batteries. There is no "magic number" for how much sleep we each need. That amount varies based on age, lifestyle, culture, health and personal needs. To keep your brain healthy and free of toxins, get seven to eight hours of sleep a night if at all possible—no less than six hours—consistently. Sleeping too much (nine hours or

more) is also associated with greater illness and accidents, so don't go overboard. Some people need more, others less. Know yourself and pay attention to your own individual needs.

Adopt a lifestyle (travel, social life and work) that lets you get enough rest. We've all mastered the process of recharging our computers, tablets, phones and devices before they run out of juice. We keep spare chargers and use airport charging stations so we're never without power. Let's become equally skilled at recharging our *human* batteries before they, too, run out.

Serena Williams is one of the greatest female tennis players in history—and one of the most recognizable names in the world. She overcame insurmountable odds to win 17 career Grand Slams and earn gold medals at the 2000, 2008 and 2012 Olympics—but she's struggled with sleeping issues for years. This struggle led her to help develop Sleep Sheets, sleep-aid strips that melt in your mouth and contain small amounts of the hormone melatonin. Melatonin is typically used to reset the body's clock after jet lag or an irregular work or personal schedule. Sleep Sheets help Williams get a good night's sleep so she wakes up each morning feeling refreshed and ready to start her day.

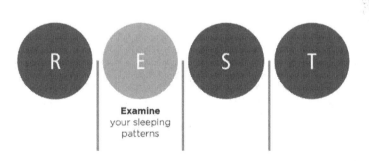

Examine
your sleeping
patterns

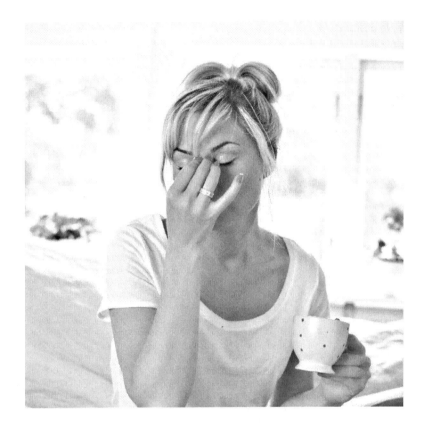

2. Examine your sleeping patterns. You can use a range of devices to monitor your sleep patterns and make sure you're getting the rest you need. Smart sleep systems that connect to mattresses or pillowcases, wearable sleep-monitoring technology, Smartphone apps and devices like Jawbone Up, Sleep Cycle, Sleepbot and Fitbit monitor your sleep quantity and quality.

Systems like SleepIQ™ have sensors built inside the bed to measure breathing rate, heart rate and movement. These innovative systems collect your sleep data and present it in easy-to-understand graphs to help you sort out the root causes of sleep issues. Some of these sleep-monitoring tools have built-in environmental sensors to track ambient light, sound, humidity, dust, pollen and temperature to identify a range of potential sleep disturbances. They can help diagnose sleep disorders you might not otherwise know about, like sleep apnea. Some devices have auto-record-ing capabilities so you can find out if you snore, talk in your sleep or have breathing problems. They also warn you if you're running on a sleep defi-cit and need to get back into a regular sleeping pattern. Be careful, though: some of these apps run on devices like Smartphones that might also inter-fere with your sleep!

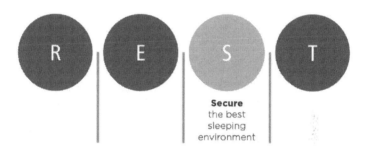

Secure
the best
sleeping
environment

3. **S**ecure the best sleeping environment. Make your room a peaceful sanctuary. For restful sleep, make sure your room is cool but not cold (60-67 degrees) to allow for the usual nighttime lowering of your body temperature. It's not always easy, but minimize light and noise as much as possible—and get help for that significant other who snores. Consider using earplugs, fans or "white noise" machines. Invest in a comfortable bed with a mattress, sheets, blankets, comforters and pil-lows that fit your needs.

You spend a large part of your day in bed (a third of it, ideally), so don't try a save a buck by getting a cheap bed. If you're using an innerspring mattress or disagree with your significant other on proper mattress firmness, consider high-end mattresses like Sleep Number® that are clinically proven to relieve back pain and improve sleep quality, but can also be adjusted to your own personal comfort. No matter what you choose to use, replace your mattress frequently enough: the average lifespan of a good-quality mattress is 9-10 years.

But a good night's sleep involves more than just your bedroom setup—it starts with decisions you make throughout the day. Try to have a consistent sleep-and- wake schedule. Seek as much light exposure in the morning as possible; this helps regulate your biological clock and keeps you in sync with the ebb and flow of the day. Try not to drink caffeine or alcohol too late in the day, since both stay in your body for hours after consumption. And finish eating at least 2-3 hours before your regular bedtime.

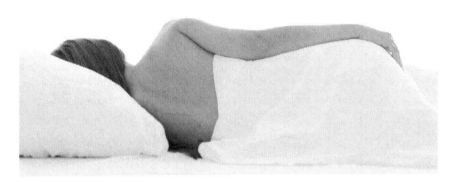

Cultivate a regular, relaxing bedtime routine— practice yoga, read a book, soak in a hot bath or listen to soothing music—to relax your body and prepare you for sleep. Experts recommend starting a bedtime routine an hour or more before you expect to fall asleep. Consider drinking caffeine-free herbal teas like jasmine and chamomile, which have calming effects. Certain smells may help, too: lavender decreases heart rate and blood pressure, and puts you in a more relaxed state.

If you're looking for best sleep practices, visit the National Sleep Foundation's website. The site helps you create the best sleep environment and shows you how to "design a sensible bedroom." It offers recommendations, research and stats about how our senses (touch, sight, hearing, smell and taste) impact sleep.

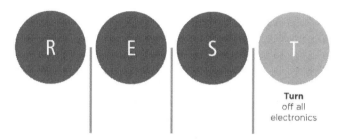

Turn
off all
electronics

4. Turn off all electronics. Have you ever gone to bed to check email or watch a show before turning off the lights after a long day? We've all been guilty of this at some point. In our 24/7 society, too many people bring their favorite gadgets into the bedroom to watch a late movie, check the news or play one last game before bedtime. But strong scientific data shows that even small electronic devices emit enough light to tease the brain and promote wakefulness. There have also been cases of phones or electrical devices accidently catching fire. So turn off all devices—TV, phone, computers and tablets—and keep them out of your bedroom altogether.

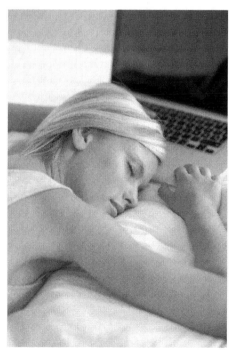

Stress is the main contributor to short-term sleeping difficulties. So aside from electronics, avoid stressful conversations and over-stimulating your mind before bedtime: it's a recipe for a sleepless night. Your brain needs to associate your bedroom with a peaceful, safe, quiet place to rest and refuel.

Sleep hygiene is critical to a healthy lifestyle, yet we tend to value it significantly less than nutrition and exercise. Sadly, we often pride ourselves on needing little sleep to function. We bend the rules, cutting into sleep time by catching an early train or a red-eye flight, going to bed late to finish a work project, or prying ourselves out of bed early so we can run errands or accomplish tasks we can't fit into a regular day. We feel exhausted, we get impatient and we can't think clearly.

> *"I exercise 2 to 3 times a week. I practice Yoga once a week. And I make sure to get plenty of sleep. I give myself 7 to 8 hours of sleep a day."*
>
> *Melanie Kannokada*

We forget that sleep is an absolute biological necessity. Studies have shown that our health is impacted when we take these kinds of short cuts, and we pay the price down the road. By contrast, getting *enough* quality sleep has amazing health benefits including improved concentration, mood, productivity and memory. So don't mess with sleep—start making it a higher priority. Jump into bed earlier at night and sleep longer hours—not just on weekends but every day of the week. Give your body the rest it needs and deserves!

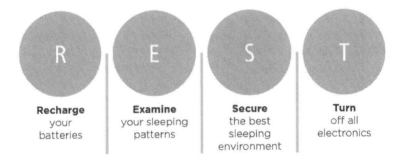

R	E	S	T
Recharge your batteries	**Examine** your sleeping patterns	**Secure** the best sleeping environment	**Turn** off all electronics

REPAIR

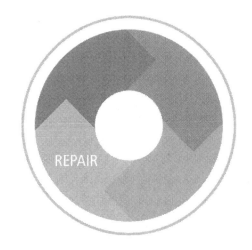

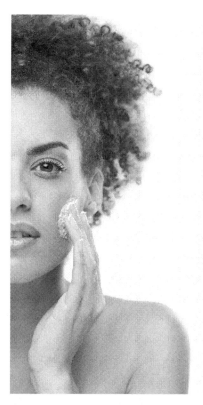

A healthy lifestyle keeps you energized; it also leads to radiant skin and a strong body. Creams, foundations, powders, eye shadows, blushes, lipsticks, perfumes and nail polish—just to name a few—have become part of a daily ritual for many women. Although they're not always necessary, when a woman uses cosmetics, she's simply enhancing what's beautiful about her. But how do women keep their skin young, fresh and glowing? Good skincare and healthy lifestyle choices—like eating well, exercising regularly and sleeping enough—can help delay the natural aging process and prevent a range of skin problems. Here are some best practices you can adopt to REPAIR and maintain healthy skin:

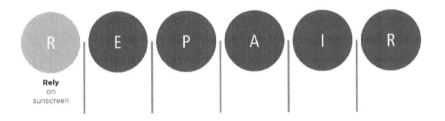

Rely
on
sunscreen

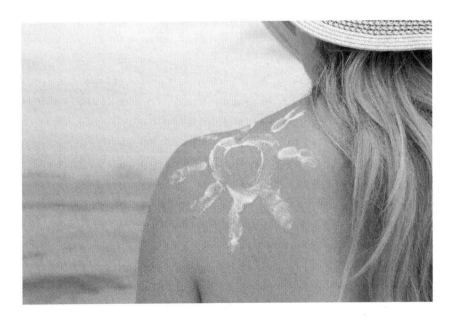

> *"Trust me. Getting a facial every two weeks makes a huge difference for your skin!"*
>
> *- Brittany Dawn Brannon*

1. **R**ely on sunscreen. One of the most important ways to take care of your skin is to protect it from the sun. A daily dose of sunscreen helps prevent skin cancer, wrinkles and sunburn, and can reduce skin aging. Too much sun exposure is known to cause long-lasting damage to the skin. Daily use of a broad-spectrum (UVA/UVB) sunscreen, SPF 15 or higher, is highly recommended. For extended outdoor activity, a water-resistant or sweat-proof, broad-spectrum (UVA/UVB) sunscreen with an SPF of 30 or higher is the way to go. Apply it evenly to all exposed skin—yes, that includes lips, ears, neck, scalp, hands, and feet—30 minutes before any outdoor activities. Reapply every two hours—or immediately after exercising or swimming, as it may have worn off. Needless to say, stay away from indoor UV-tanning salons: studies show that tanning bed use increases the risk of melanoma, a form of skin cancer that can be deadly.

> *"I am a big fan of encouraging women to look natural. Don't show too much. Stay classy at all times."*
>
> *- Connor Boss*

Allyson Felix is a track-and-field sprint athlete and a U.S. Olympic sprinter. Her accomplishments include a gold medal in the 4 x 400 relay at the Beijing games and two Olympic silver medals in the 200m. She's also an eight-time world champion. Off the track, she's an ambassador for the President's Council on Fitness, Sports & Nutrition. She describes herself as "Christian. Pinkberry Lover. Self-proclaimed fashionista. Family Girl. Insanely Competitive. Kind of Silly. Always ready to race whoever, whenever to the light post and back." Felix also knows how to care for her skin and enjoy cosmetic products. She uses a daily moisturizer with SPF 30 to keeps her skin hydrated and protected at all times: "This works great for me during the day because it's very hydrating and protects my skin from the sun when I'm on the track," she told Beauty.com.

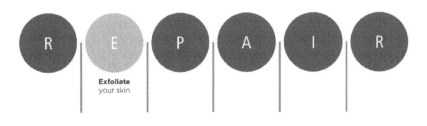

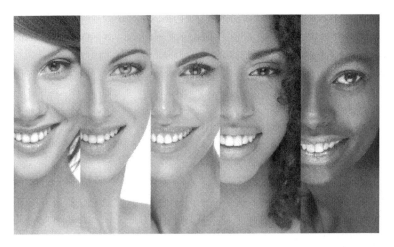

2. **E**xfoliate your skin. Exfoliation should be part of anyone's weekly skin-care routine to remove dead skin cells and generate collagen. Find the right balance: scrubbing too rarely, too little or too lightly won't give you the benefits you want from a good exfoliation routine; scrubbing too much, too often or too hard can damage your skin. You have many exfoliation options: facial scrubs, washcloths, microdermabrasion, chemical peels, or retinoids. Pick what works best for you. If you have dry skin after you exfoliate, try extra-virgin coconut oil or a similar product to keep your skin moisturized. See what Unilever recommends in the "Did You Know" section called "10 Tips For Even More Beautiful Skin."

R E P A I R

Pamper
hands and feet

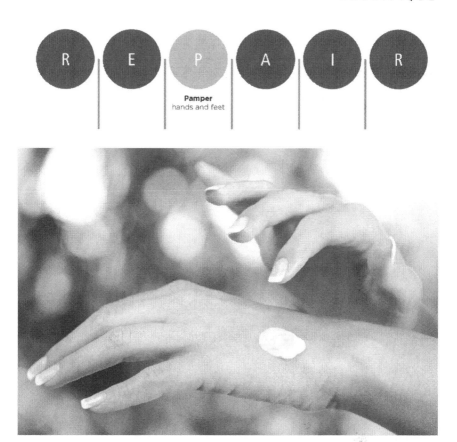

3. **P**amper your hands and feet. Like your face, both hands and feet get regular exposure to the elements, so they need extra care and attention. Visible skin changes attributed to aging— which show up on your hands as wrinkles, brown spots and leathery skin—are caused by the sun's UV radiation. Hands and feet are also prone to dryness because of frequent hand washing and the skin's natural thinness in these areas. Consider using a moisturizing sunscreen with an SPF of 15 or higher, with antioxidants such as vitamin C or E. Keep some on hand in convenient places: not just the bathroom, but also your kitchen, bedroom, office and even your car. Apply regularly to keep your hands and feet hydrated, protected and healthy looking.

> *"As women, we need to feel beautiful. We like putting a dress on, fixing our hair and putting make up on. It feels great and we should celebrate that."*
>
> *- Marika Siewert*

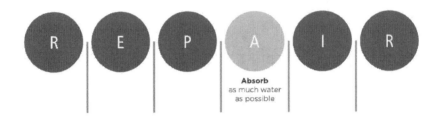

Absorb
as much water
as possible

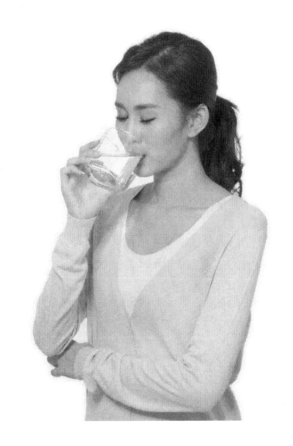

4. **A**bsorb as much water as possible. Getting enough water every day is vital to your health. Water is actually your body's main chemical component—it makes up sixty percent of your body weight! There's no single formula; the right amount of water intake varies based on your health, activity level and environment. In a temperate climate, the adequate liquid intake for women is 2.2 liters per day. Thankfully, you meet most of your fluid needs through the water and beverages you drink. But you can also get fluids through the foods you eat— especially foods with high water content, like tomatoes or cucumbers. Because our bodies can't always tell whether we're hungry or thirsty, next time you feel like grabbing a snack, try drinking a full glass of water instead. A study found that people who drank water before meals ate fewer calories at each meal. Drinking water is essential to keeping your body well fueled. Drinking lots of water—six to eight glasses a day—will flush your body of toxins and make your skin look more radiant.

Christie Brinkley is one of America's most successful and recognizable models. Since the mid-1970s, she's appeared on over 500 magazine covers worldwide, and she's been the face of many major brands. Born in 1954, the artist, writer, designer, actress and political activist holds the longest-running cosmetics contract of any model in history. Brinkley still looks amazing— look her up online. Her glowing, youthful appearance remains her unique trademark. When asked about her beauty secrets, she confessed, "My routine is very simple: I cleanse, exfoliate, and moisturize." Proper hydration is key to her vitality and ageless beauty: "I also drink tons of water to keep my skin hydrated." It seems that water—not diamonds—is a girl's best friend.

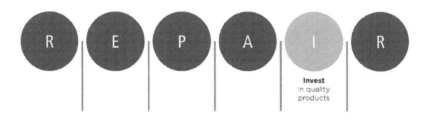

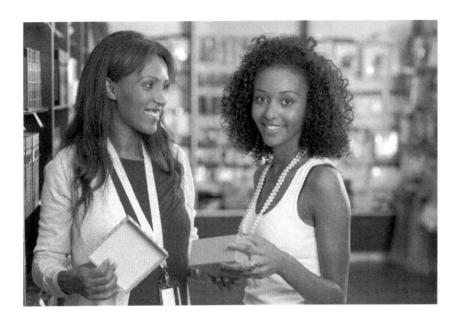

5. **I**nvest in quality products. Given that your skin is the body's largest organ, a good moisturizer is essential, and vital to keeping your skin balanced. Buy quality skincare products with healthy ingredients. It's tempting to fill your shopping cart with cheap or "on-sale" skincare products that may not be the right products for you. Go beyond the clever and sometimes confusing marketing claims and read labels carefully before you buy. You'll be surprised to learn what's included. Some of the ingredients might dry your skin, or you might be sensitive to a particular product. Whatever goes on your skin goes inside your body—so be selective. It's not always easy, though. Take mineral oil, a common ingredient in lip balms and moisturizers: some experts consider it undesirable, while others say it's perfectly safe. You'll need to decide for yourself. Thankfully, there are alternatives if you're concerned about potential health risks. Sample products before buying to find the right match. Visit stores like Sephora or Nordstrom to seek help and guidance from informed sales associates. If you are what you eat, you are also what you put on your body. Not unlike food and sleep, skincare is not an area where you want to save a buck.

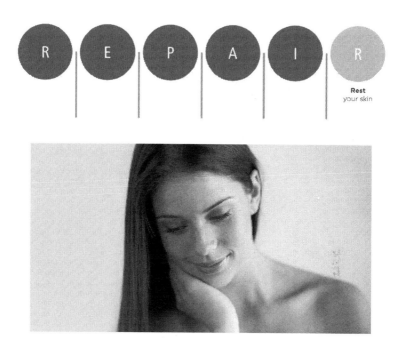

R E P A I R

Rest
your skin

6. **R**est your skin. Your body needs rest, and so does your skin. Every day, dirt, dust and sun exposure all contribute to damaging your skin over time. If you have an active lifestyle, you may get your skin scratched or damaged even more quickly, so take action to minimize the impact. Find a good cleanser that your skin responds well to. Be careful not to over-cleanse your skin. Consider paring down your makeup routine to expose your pores to more oxygen: rashes and breakouts will be less likely.

Greek-American actress, TV host and journalist Maria Menounos has become a familiar face to many. Her appearances have ranged from reporting on the *NBC Nightly News* to competing on *Dancing with the Stars*. In her book *The Everygirl's Guide to Life,* Menounos (known for her gorgeous skin) says that one of the first steps to great skin is a healthy skincare routine. "My main thing is that I make sure I wash my face every night, no matter what." She adds,

I even do a white glove test to make sure it's all off. . . . My other trick is that I use one white face towel and then put it the hamper. I use a clean towel every time I wash. Just never re-use towels, they have all that bacteria!

Menounos knows too well that to get amazing results, you must give your skin the rest it so badly needs.

Protect and nurture your skin as if it's your most precious asset. Sun protection is essential to skincare and cancer prevention, as skin damage occurs with each unprotected exposure and accumulates over the course of your lifetime. It's a lifelong journey and a year-round commitment to give your skin the best chance for long-term health and beauty. Organizations like the Skin Cancer Foundation offer a number of great recommendations. If you're looking for a checklist, consider Unilever's ten principles of optimum skincare.

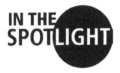

IN THE SPOTLIGHT

10 Tips For Even More Beautiful Skin

1. Scrub the right way. Extremes are bad for your skin. Scrubbing too little will leave you looking dull; too much is, well, too much. Use a mild exfoliating product (avoid ingredients like almond shells, which can be rough on skin). And resist the temptation to scrub too hard: a gentle massage is all it takes to remove makeup and dead skin cells and improve circulation.

2. Seal in the good stuff. The best time to moisturize is when skin still feels damp—the moisturizer will act as a sealant and help hydrate your skin. So start a habit of moisturizing every time you bathe, shower or even wash your hands.

3. Use sunblock—from head to toe. Many people think that basking on the beach for days on end is what causes skin cancer. In fact, the short sun exposure you get every day can also put you at risk. Use a moisturizer that contains both UVA and UVB protection, and be sure to cover all exposed areas, including hands, forearms, face and ears.

4. Pamper your hands and feet. Your hands are continually exposed to sun and are one of the first areas to show environmental damage. Be sure to wash your hands with a mild cleanser like Dove Cream Bar, followed by moisturizer. To soothe dry, rough feet, slather on a rich moisturizer at bedtime and slip on a pair of socks for intense healing while you sleep.

5. Plan your next trip. Before stepping on an airplane, drench your skin with moisturizing products since re-circulated air tends to dry skin out. And don't forget to buy a bottle of water (or two) for the flight after you've made it past security.

6. Don't be water-resistant. While drinking water won't directly moisturize your skin, it will help your internal organs function properly, which affects your skin's health and beauty. Ditto with exercise.

7. Find the fat. We're talking mono-unsaturated fats here, found in nuts and olive, canola and safflower oils. It's easy to incorporate these fats (which are low in saturated fats) into your daily diet. One tablespoon of oil, a quarter cup of nuts or two tablespoons of peanut butter will do the trick.

8. Water your air. Just as winter air wreaks havoc on your skin, so does your summer air conditioner. Counteract the drying effects with a humidifier, which puts water back into the air and helps your skin stay moisturized. Well-hydrated skin looks plumper and more youthful.

9. Be a sleeping beauty. Your skin reflects your mental and physical condition, so skimping on shut-eye results in sallowness and more noticeable wrinkles. Listen to doctors—they recommend eight hours a night.

10. Take a break. A high stress level is bad for your mood and your skin. Treat yourself to at least one relaxing, pampering activity per week, be it a bubble bath flanked by candles, a facial or a movie marathon at home.

Courtesy of Unilever

Of course, there's nothing like happiness to make your skin glow—add some spice to your life and see what it does to your skin!

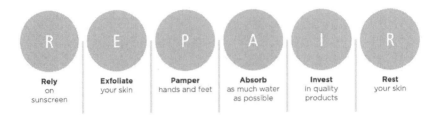

Rely	Exfoliate	Pamper	Absorb	Invest	Rest
on sunscreen	your skin	hands and feet	as much water as possible	in quality products	your skin

Feeling good and bringing out your best physical self help build self-esteem and confidence. Taking care of your body and your appearance are essential responsibilities in pursuing inner and outer beauty. Eating wisely, exercising regularly, sleeping enough and nurturing your skin are essential to a healthy lifestyle. Follow the principles we reviewed in this chapter (and summarized below) and you'll be well underway to feeling amazing:

> *"Women are hard on themselves. We strive to have it all and sometimes we fall below our own expectations. It's not unusual to focus on the things we don't have like beauty, relationships, etc. Yet each of us carries special beauty that no one else has."*
>
> *- Maureen Francisco*

Fuel	Burn	Rest	Repair
Forget fake and highly processed food	Break up your workout routine	Recharge your batteries	Rely on sun screen
Use the right nutrients	Unleash the fun	Examine your sleeping patterns	Exfoliate your skin
Evaluate the calories you consume	Reach your weekly goals	Secure the best sleeping environment	Pamper hands & feet
Lower your sugar intake	Nourish the practice of walking everywhere	Turn off all electronics	Absorb as much water as possible
			Invest in quality products
			Rest your skin

Although all four best practices (Fuel–Burn–Rest–Repair) are essential to a strong and healthy body, we each may value or emphasize them differently. In other words, some may focus on areas they feel deserve greater effort and attention, less on other areas. In a study I conducted with Google Consumer Services, I discovered that most women value eating smart (Fuel), exercising (Burn), followed by getting sleep (Rest) and skincare (Repair). Every woman must find the right balance to satisfy her own personal needs at each particular moment.

IN YOUR OPINION, WHAT CONTRIBUTES TO A
STRONG, HEALTHY BODY?

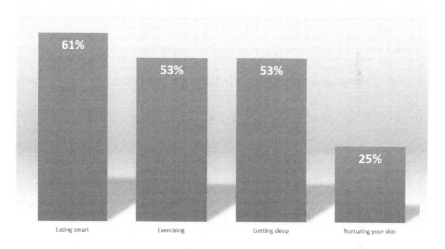

No matter what choices you make, remember that each habit enhances the others: exercise more and you'll likely sleep better. Make healthy choices a priority in your busy life. Feeling healthy— and happy about our appearance—is all we can ask of ourselves. We can learn to love our bodies and ourselves by becoming aware of the incredible diversity of human shapes and sizes among us.

Accepting your body is accepting yourself. If you feel great, you also look great. Hope Solo would agree.

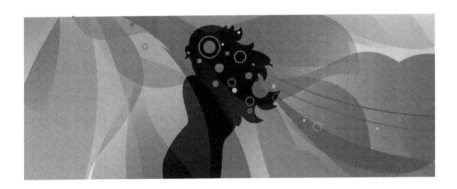

*"Usually, when people say
you are beautiful,
it is when there is a harmony
between the inside and the outside."*

**- Emmanuel Beart,
French actress and César Award winner**

CHAPTER FIVE
THE BEAUTIFUL
AND OPEN MIND

It was in the bathroom that Sara Blakely turned her dream and $5,000 life savings into $1 billion. The woman that many women thank for trimming their curves and boosting their bottoms managed to convince a Neiman Marcus buyer to follow her to the ladies' room, where she personally demonstrated the benefits of her product.

Blakely's story is no ordinary one. Although she initially wanted to become an attorney, her LSAT scores forced her to reconsider her career goals. After a short stint at Walt Disney World she joined an office supply company to sell fax machines; the job required her to wear pantyhose in the hot and humid Florida weather. She started a multi-billion-dollar business by simply cutting the feet out of control-top pantyhose. The look of a seamed foot with open-toed shoes bothered her, but she enjoyed the firmer look and the eliminated panty lines that the control top offered.

A few weeks after the meeting that ended in the ladies' room, Sara's first SPANX product appeared on the selective shelves of Neiman Marcus. Next came Nordstrom, Saks and many other fine boutiques, upscale department stores and major retail chains like Target. SPANX ended up being featured on *The Oprah Winfrey Show, The Today Show* and CNN, and in major magazines and newspapers from *Vogue* to the *New York Times*. The product became a huge success and a red-carpet must for celebrities like Gwyneth Paltrow. In 2001, Blakely sold 8,000 pairs in the first six minutes on the home-shopping channel QVC.

Blakely's lack of business experience didn't get in the way of her ambitions. In an interview with CNBC, she admitted, "I had never taken a business class, had no training, didn't know how retail worked. I wasn't as intimidated as I should have been." She added, "What you don't know can become your greatest asset if you'll let it, and if you have the confidence to say, I'm going to do it anyway." After coming up with her idea she taught herself about trademarks and patents, poring over specialized books for weeks. With only a modest $5,000 investment she couldn't afford an attorney, so she wrote the patent herself. Finding a manufacturer required the same perseverance; she did online research on hosiery manufacturers for months before contacting them.

Another important lesson from Blakely's success story is her ability to learn from mistakes. Each day when she was young, her father would ask, "So, what did you fail at lately?" His encouragement to learn through failure gave her an entrepreneurial spirit and the courage to follow her heart without fear—a trait that's critical to her success. Blakely's mom offered support too. A comedian at heart, she jokes that "mom always said as long as I lifted my pants up and not down to show my product then I had her blessing!"

A strong mind in a strong body is the ultimate advantage. As Blakely proved, if we condition our mind properly, we can accomplish anything we set out to do. Getting there can be tricky, though. There's plenty of expert advice on how to build a strong body; resources on building a strong mind are a bit harder to come by. Neuroscience (the study of the nervous system) and cognitive psychology (the study of mental processes) are both grounded in the quest to better understand the brain and the role of memory, perception, creativity, problem solving and thinking.

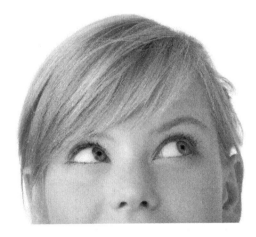

We're all different in our ability to think. A popular method for assessing this skill is known as IQ ("intelligence quotient"), a score derived from one of several standardized tests designed to assess intelligence. Alfred Binet, a French psychologist, developed the test on which today's IQ tests are based. Binet's test aimed to predict a student's chance of success by focusing on topics outside the usual school curriculum: memory, attention and basic problem-solving skills. Although we're all born with certain mental abilities, we can further develop and enhance them during our lifetime.

We ask ourselves: How do I build brainpower? How do I improve my mental abilities? How can I unlock my mind's full potential? Sure, there are countless memory-building, problem-solving exercises, puzzles and other techniques to build a stronger, more effective mind. But I believe that a beautiful and open mind is based on four main competencies, as illustrated below in the "Mind Journey Wheel of Success":

- **LISTEN:** our capacity to listening well
- **LEARN:** our aptitude for learning from our successes and mistakes, and from others
- **CONNECT:** our ability to stay well informed on what's happening in the world and in our community
- **MASTER:** our capability to express ourselves effectively by mastering verbal and written communication.

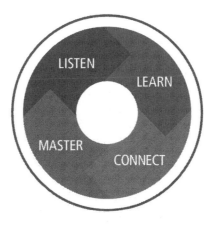

Figure 1 Mind Journey Wheel of Success

Once these skills are fully developed, your mind is far clearer, stronger and more focused—and it comes across that way to others. It's the careful combination of these mental competencies that unlocks your potential and makes you shine. Let's take a more careful look at each competency, exploring what it's made of and how you can apply it in everyday life:

LISTEN

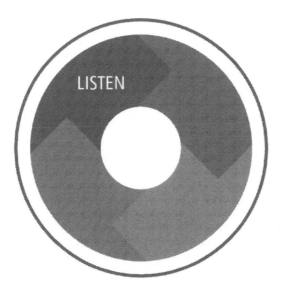

In today's high-speed environment, communication is more important than ever. Yet we devote little time and effort to master communication skills that can help us build stronger relationships, solve problems and improve our interactions with others.

Let's start with listening. Most of us take our hearing ability for granted. For Joanne Milne, hearing means something quite special. She was born deaf due to Usher syndrome, a genetic condition that causes hearing loss. At the age of 39, Milne was fitted with two cochlear implants (surgically implanted electronic devices that improve hearing by stimulating the auditory nerve). After the surgery she burst into tears when she heard a nurse reading out the days of the week; the moment was captured on video and went viral. Milne put it this way: "Hearing things for the first time is so, so emotional, from the ping of a light switch to running water. I can't stop crying."

> *"If I had to start over, I would take time to make my decisions. In the end, I am the only one in charge of what happens to me. I learned not to be afraid of asking questions so I can make better informed decisions."*
>
> *- Marika Siewert*

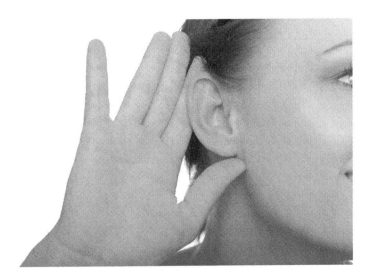

Those of us who are blessed with functional hearing need to reacquaint ourselves with this gift of nature. To hear is to perceive with our ears what someone says to us. To *listen* is to pay attention with our other senses— and our whole brain— to help us fully understand the words being spoken. We hear with our auditory system, of course, and we listen to make sense of messages using our main cognitive functions: attention, memory and reason.

Listening is one of the important skills you can develop to improve your understanding of others. At work, listening well means reading people's signs and taking into consideration what others say; it'll make you a better co-worker, manager or employee. At home, listening well means relating better to those you love, understanding them better; it'll help you become more supportive of them. Everywhere else, listening well means building friendships and becoming connected to our community.

"When you are asked a difficult or controversial question, go with your feelings and follow your instincts. If you speak from the heart, you will capture people's hearts and attention."

- Kristen Dalton

But listening well isn't easy, given that most of us only retain a small amount of what's shared with us verbally—this often leads to painful misunderstandings and unnecessary conflicts. We may be quick to interrupt others while they are still speaking, correct their facts, share our perspective and enlighten the world with our great wisdom. We feel justified in doing so. Unfortunately, our own beliefs and opinions keep us from fully understanding what the other person is saying.

We often fail to practice the art of active listening. Active listening is a mindset, an approach to more careful listening that goes beyond the words themselves, recognizing non-verbal cues and body language. Percussionist and composer Evelyn Glennie lost nearly all her hearing by age 12. This condition didn't discourage her from pursuing her love for music. In her 2003 TED Talk called "How to Truly Listen," Glennie explains that she can hear music through her hands, arms, cheekbones, scalp, abdomen, chest, legs and every part of her body.

To truly hear we must depend on much more than simply the ear, which can be easily misled by the room we're in, amplification, instrument quality and more. Listening well requires our full and undivided attention, focusing on truly understanding what's being said and why, instead of planning what to say next or forming a counter argument. It requires setting aside our own personal or cultural filters that can alter how we interpret someone's message. It requires acknowledging, validating and precise questioning to make sure we're not leaping to assumptions.

Our ability to listen affects our ability to understand situations, learn, make decisions, feel empathy, influence others, be productive and build relationships. We tend to talk too much and listen too little. The Greek philosopher Epictetus' saying, "We have two ears and one mouth so that we can listen twice as much as we speak," makes clear what we should be doing instead.

> *"My iPad keeps me updated on news, keeps me organized. I have access to all of my favorite books with the iBook app. I can network with my peers. And there's practically an app for everything, which makes my life much easier!"*
>
> *- Heidi Forrest*

Active listening has a huge impact on how we consume and digest information. This translates into deeper insights, better decisions, richer relationships and more effective communication in general. Here's more on how to LISTEN.

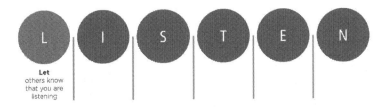

Let others know that you are listening

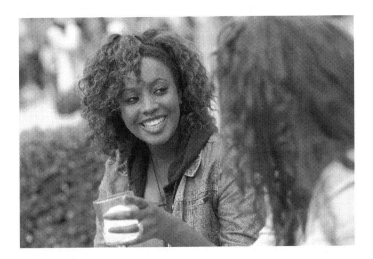

1. Let others know you're listening. Show them that you hear what they're saying, that you're interested and genuinely want to understand their perspective. Don't interrupt them. Let them finish their thoughts—even though you think you've figured out what they'll say next. You may have, but finishing people's sentences has never proven helpful at building a better dialogue. Be patient. Provide ongoing acknowledgment and feedback, either verbally or physically (nod your head, smile, maintain eye contact, keep an open posture, limit your movements and say things like "I hear you" or "I understand"). People open up and speak more freely when we show them our full attention.

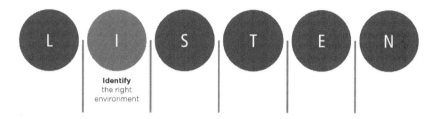

L I S T E N

Identify
the right
environment

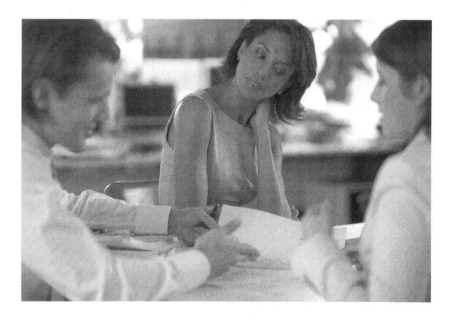

2. **I**dentify the right environment. Pick the right place to have a conversation so you can be attentive—a quiet, inviting room. A quality conversation is more likely to happen in a relaxing, neutral, calm environment. People tend to speak more slowly in a friendly environment. Where would you rather negotiate a new contract or take someone one a date? In a stressful, noisy environment, we rush to get to the point. Avoid distractions or multi-tasking so you can stay alert and engaged in the entire conversation. Keep in mind that you're listening for both *what's* being said and *how*. *Where* it's being said also sets the tone and influences your discussion.

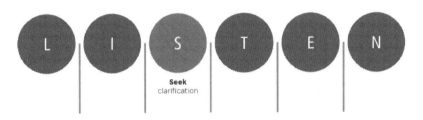

3. **S**eek clarification. We often hear what we want to hear. Ask questions so nothing's open to interpretation or subject to bias or opinions ("What do you mean by that?" or "Am I understanding you correctly when you say that . . . ?"). Ask questions that move the conversation forward and further your understanding. If you're not sure, summarize what you've heard to confirm your understanding and give others a chance to provide more information. In my career, I've been amazed at answers I received from a conversation I thought I fully understood—but clearly missed some critical information along the way or misinterpreted what was said. It's important to ensure clarity and agreement.

> *"Listen carefully. You will learn
> some life-long interpersonal
> success skills that classrooms
> can't and won't teach you."*
>
> *- Maureen Francisco*

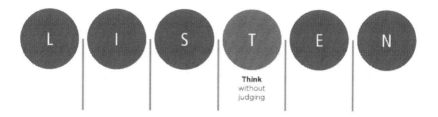

Think
without
judging

4.   Think without judging. Keep an open mind and listen carefully without jumping to premature conclusions. Reflect on what the other person is saying before you respond. Don't let your own thoughts or biases distract you.

Michelle Kwan, five-time world champion figure skater and two-time Olympic medalist, knows a thing or two about listening with an open mind. The most-decorated figure skater in U.S. history began skating at age five. She entered and won her first figure-skating competition a year later. The daughter of Hong Kong immigrants, Kwan quickly learned that hard work, great listening skills and an open mind are essential to success. Kwan listened to many coaches during her career to improve her staking techniques, leading her to an amazing career. In 2006, she was named a public diplomacy ambassador representing American values around the world, listening and discovering values from other countries, from Russia and China to Ukraine and South Korea. While Kwan may have a "heart of a champion" (the title of her autobiography), her many accomplishments remind us of her ability to listen well, learn quickly and keep an open mind.

> *"A woman's mindset will either limit or launch her into seeing her own beauty and potential. She will only attain what her perceived potential is. The way a woman thinks, whether positive, negative or indifferent, will become her reality."*
>
> *- Maureen Francisco*

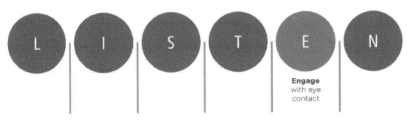

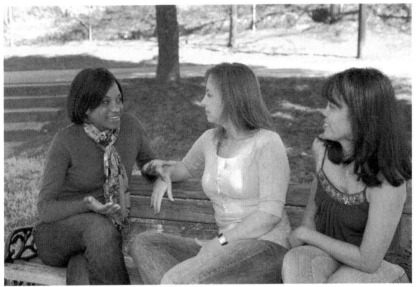

5. **E**ngage with eye contact. Do you always face the person talking to you, maintaining eye contact? In a multi-tasking culture where we feel justified checking countless SMS or instant Facebook messages coming in rapid fire, we need to make an extra effort to remind ourselves of simple yet important behaviors like eye contact. When you do, you show that you care about what's being said, and you actively engage in the conversation. You can also read situations and interpret people better.

Consider the most famous softball pitcher of her era: Jennie Finch. How could you not make eye contact with a woman who has a cannon for an arm? Knowing that Finch's pitches top out at 72 miles per hour, you wouldn't want to look anywhere else but right at her eyes! An ambassador for both softball and for female athletes in general, Finch started pitching when she was eight years old; she won many competitions, including a gold medal at the Athens Summer Olympics. She pitched for the Arizona Wildcats, the USA national softball team and the Chicago Bandits.

> *"Beauty comes from within. It's not about physical beauty but rather about what you project."*
>
> *- Connor Boss*

You don't need to play softball to know to look someone in the eyes. But next time you need to maintain eye contact with someone, imagine Jennie Finch throwing a ball at you. It does the trick for me every time.

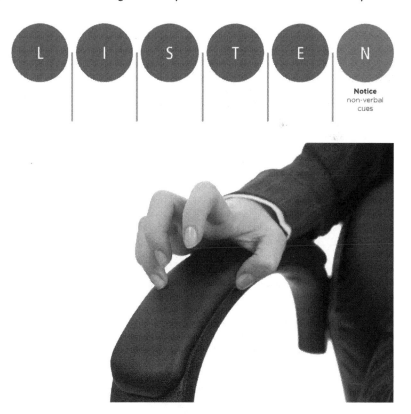

L I S T E N

Notice
non-verbal
cues

6. **N**otice non-verbal cues. Have you ever watched a politician give a speech with the television on mute? A foreign film without subtitles? It's amazing how much we can learn from non-verbal cues. Look for signs like facial expressions and body posture. Are they closing their arms while speaking, perhaps showing disagreement or unwillingness to reconsider their position? Are they playing nervously with their hands, showing impatience or disapproval? Do they appear to move their body towards you and away from you?

The majority of our direct communication is non-verbal. Most of us could watch a play with earplugs and still understand it just by watching the actors' movement and expressions. We learned to read these cues instinctively in childhood, and often take them for granted. We need to pay closer attention to what others say to us, even unconsciously. Our eyes, mouth, hands and shoulders simply speak louder than words.

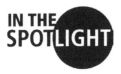

IN THE SPOTLIGHT

Basic Listening Skills Test

Do you practice active listening in everyday situations? Here's a quick way to check. Answer the following questions:

1. Do you often stop someone in mid-sentence to interject your opinion if you disagree with a statement he/she's made, or if you have something to add to the conversation?

2. While someone is talking, do you find yourself thinking about what you're going to say next?

3. Do you show signs of impatience or feel like finishing someone's sentences while he/she's speaking to you?

---

4. Do you find yourself checking your phone or your watch when someone's speaking to you?

5. Do you feel impatient when someone isn't getting straight to the point?

6. When listening to someone, do you always make and maintain eye contact?

7. When you agree with what someone's saying, do you occasionally nod your head?

8. If you're unsure whether you've grasped someone's point correctly, do you summarize your understanding of what he/she said to confirm that you've got it right?

9. Do you feel like you're giving your full attention and avoiding distractions (like looking around or listening to another conversation) when someone's speaking to you?

10. Do you ask questions to encourage someone to elaborate on his/her point?

11. Do you wait for someone to finish her point before making a mental judgment on what he/she said?

12. When listening to someone speaking, do you pay close attention to his/her body language?

If you answered "yes" to questions 1-5 and "no" to questions 6-12, practicing active listening with a friend or family member to improve your skills. Make note of these 12 typical listening behaviors, follow best practices in active listening (questions 6-12) and avoid common traps (questions 1-5).

Julian Treasure is chair of the Sound Agency, a firm that advises businesses on how to use sound. He spoke at TEDGlobal in 2011 on "five ways to listen better." Treasure claims that "we are losing our listening. We spend roughly 60 percent of our communication time listening, but we're not very good at it. We retain just 25 percent of what we hear." Why? A range of filters—culture, language, values, attitudes and expectations—get in the way. Those who listen well learn faster and connect better than others.

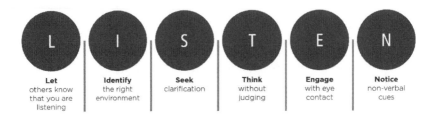

Let	**Identify**	**Seek**	**Think**	**Engage**	**Notice**
others know that you are listening	the right environment	clarification	without judging	with eye contact	non-verbal cues

LEARN

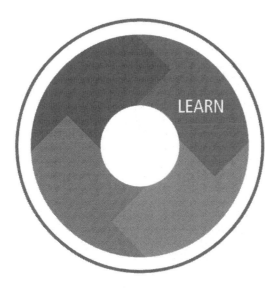

How we learn varies significantly from individual to individual. We learn from the day we're born—it's central to our ability to survive and thrive. We learn from our experiences, good and bad: we fall from our bikes, scratch our knees, get our hearts broken.

According to right-brain/left-brain theory, we use both sides of our brain to think and learn. As individuals, our capacity to learn appears limitless. When we're young, our brain acts as a sponge, absorbing endless information we're exposed to. We learn from what we do well and what we could have done better. We may receive a formal education where we learn how to gather, categorize and store information for future use. The brain acts as a sort of bank where we deposit knowledge and withdraw it later to overcome challenges and pursue opportunities.

> *"I learned from my mistakes and that gave me an extra boost of confidence. I see failure as a learning experience."*
>
> *- Susie Castillo*

Learning through experience is always best. Confucius, the Chinese teacher and philosopher (551–479 BC), said, "Tell me and I will forget. Show me and I will remember. Involve me and I will understand." Our successes and mistakes become an important part of the roadmap to continued growth and development; we work to reproduce successes and avoid past mistakes.

Sometimes we have the chance to learn from other people's experiences. Eleanor Roosevelt once said, "Learn from the mistakes of others. You can't live long enough to make them all yourself." There's truth to that statement. We're conditioned to learn from early childhood from our surroundings and from other people—family and trusted friends. Yet outside of that circle, many of us won't dare ask questions or admit we lack knowledge on a particular topic. We feel embarrassed or insecure. We'd rather pretend to know something, nodding our head awkwardly. Instead, we should ask for clarification and seek to understand.

> *"The key ingredient to success, well-being and happiness is to surround yourself with positive people who will breathe wisdom and life into you versus those that drain your energy."*
>
> *- Maureen Francisco*

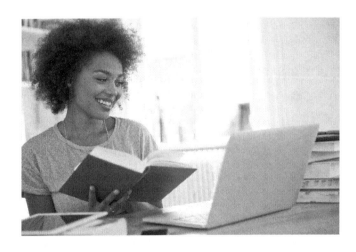

We learn from watching others, listening to them and interacting with them. We run ideas by them, seek their feedback, and ask for their perspective. We benefit from their expertise. These people may be coaches, mentors, teachers, friends or family members. Their wisdom, encouragement and words of advice shape our decisions and our perspective. Fully embrace these learning opportunities: we all need to build a support team of trusted people who give us feedback and guidance.

Learning is like a muscle—we must flex it regularly. The quicker we learn, the faster our mind can adapt to new situations and thrive. Thankfully, we have endless resources literally at our fingertips these days because of the internet—every question has an answer on Google, a blog or a website. Other rich educational resources allow us to earn degrees and attend seminars from the comfort of our own homes. Learning is a way of life we must each commit to. We can learn from everything: from every facet of life, from everyone, all the time. When we do, we open our minds to great possibilities.

> *"Confidence is key in anything you do in life. Don't let others take over your nerves. Don't freak out. Just be in the moment and be yourself at all times. In the end, you learn from every mistake. Life is about learning."*
>
> *- Heidi Forrest*

Here are some essentials to help you integrate LEARNing into your daily life:

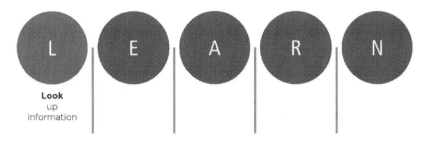

L — Look up information
E
A
R
N

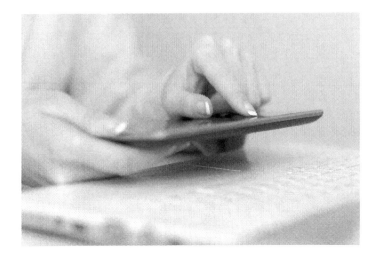

1. **L**ook up information. If you're not learning, you're not developing. Make learning a daily activity and a way of life. Information access has never been easier thanks to the rapid growth of the internet. Vast amounts of information are uploaded every day, putting a wealth of knowledge easily within your reach. Access to this sort of knowledge bank is of unprecedented scale in human history. Become a fanatic Google searcher—and have fun while you're at it! Research something you're interested in every day; look up all type of resources available at your fingertips. Make it part of your social life to quiz people and look up answers together.

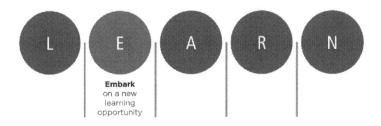

2. **E**mbark on a new learning opportunity. Consider continuing your education, no matter your age or your educational background. There's always a class, seminar or conference to attend, no matter how busy you tell yourself you are. Online education has become an incredibly rich and popular choice for anyone to take web-based classes, participate in

webinars and learn a new trade or skill set. Consider Kristen Stewart's story. The highest-paid actress in 2012, the face of Chanel and Balenciaga and the female lead in *The Twilight Saga* film series, Stewart attended school until the seventh grade. As her acting career took off, she continued her education by correspondence until she finished high school. Admired by millions of preteens, Stewart loves to read—she plans to attend college to study literature and pursue a career in writing.

> *"Success for me is progress. Each and every day I learned something. I asked myself: did I have an impact? Did I make the world a better place? Did I grow emotionally or intellectually? Making the world a better place, improving people's life, inspiring them, that's the real meaning behind working to fulfill your inner potential."*
>
> *- Melanie Kannokada*

Abraham Lincoln used to say, "Give me six hours to chop down a tree and I will spend the first four sharpening the axe." His message: preparation and learning new skills are essential to anything we do. Sharpening our axe is the equivalent of committing ourselves to learning for life.

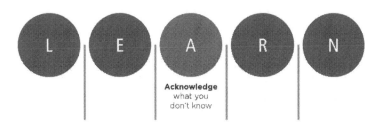

3. **A**cknowledge what you don't know. Don't pretend to know something if you don't. I met my fair share of individuals over the years, both in personal and professional settings, pretending to know more than they actually did. We sometimes feel more vulnerable when we don't know the

answer to a question. Have the courage to ask questions and you'll learn faster—soon, you may be more knowledgeable than anyone around you! When you acknowledge you don't know much about a topic, you suddenly free yourself to learn. There's something incredibly refreshing and liberating about being confident enough to admit our own limitations. Try it a few times and see how it affects your ability to learn faster.

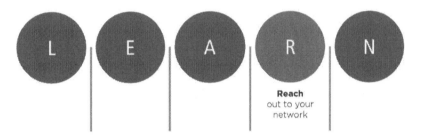

Reach
out to your
network

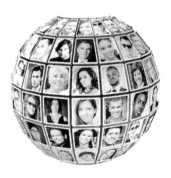

4. **R**each out to your network. Build a support team you can seek out when you have questions; you'll get advice, perspective and feedback on things that matter to you. Everyone has a network to learn from: some of us have large families, friends or colleagues. Others may have a select network of very close friends and trusted resources. Social networks like Facebook or LinkedIn also offer amazing ways to build, expand and leverage your network. No matter how big or established your network, learn to tap into it. Ask questions. Learn from others' experience. Return the favor. Oprah Winfrey suggests reaching out to a carefully assembled group of people we trust to have a good influence on us: "Surround yourself only with people who are going to take you higher."

"Surround yourself with people who love you and are an integral part of your life. No matter the outcome, they will be there to support you."

- Brittany Dawn Brannon

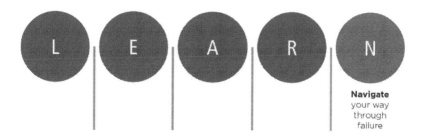

Navigate
your way
through
failure

5. **N**avigate your way through failure. Don't fear failing—it's inevitable. Make every failure a learning experience. Apply what you learn so you never repeat the same mistake twice. American actress, singer and model Scarlett Johansson began acting at a young age; she first appeared onstage on Broadway at age eight and made her film debut at nine. She had to learn early on how to cope with rejection and criticism: "I don't do damsel in distress very well. It's hard for me to play a victim." Now considered one of Hollywood's most talented actresses, the recipient of countless awards and nominations for films like *Girl with a Pearl Earring* and *Lost in Translation* learned quickly from her mistakes. Johansson knew to take responsibility for her missteps and learn from them; this ability translated into an incredibly successful career.

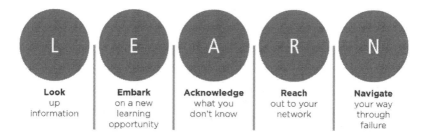

Look
up
information

Embark
on a new
learning
opportunity

Acknowledge
what you
don't know

Reach
out to your
network

Navigate
your way
through
failure

CONNECT

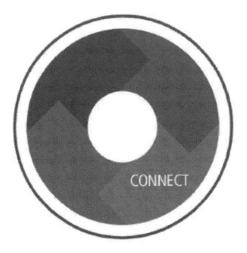

Today's world is more volatile, more complex and more interconnected than ever. Changes happening at the speed of light can transform our everyday lives. As responsible world citizens, leaders and community members, we owe ourselves to stay informed about current affairs.

Staying connected to what's going on in the world and in your local communities is the best way to be an active participant in shaping the present and future. When you do, you not only impact your personal life; you impact others' lives too. Your opinions and viewpoints suddenly matter, triggering thoughtful conversations. Being engaged improves your ability to understand others and sharpens your mind.

> *"To be successful in any environment, you need to be sharp and keep yourself well informed of current events. With the advancement of technology, people around the planet are connected 24/7. It's so easy these days with the internet. There is no excuse. Take the time to read and learn."*
>
> *- Susie Castillo*

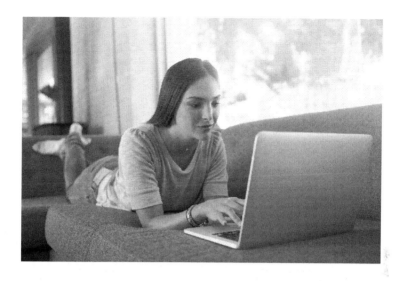

In today's technologically advanced environment, ways to stay informed have multiplied—our biggest challenge isn't to locate those resources, but to filter through the sea of information. We check the news on our smart phones and mobile devices. We rely on email, Facebook and Twitter to get last-minute updates. At this pace, relying on trustworthy, unbiased sources of information becomes critical. As we gain speed, we often lose track of fact versus opinion, and we don't always have the perspective needed to process information accurately.

Once we're in a position to receive the right information at the right time, we can form our own opinions on what it means. We develop an opinion based on information we've received, and it's shaped by our own values, judgments and experiences. We can then share that perspective with others, inviting them into an open, respectful, two-way conversation. We may agree or disagree with each other. What truly matters is *why* we do, and how we reached a particular conclusion. The goal isn't to "win" an argument, but to deepen our understanding—to open our minds to new ideas and perspectives. When we do, we make a greater contribution to the world around us. By contributing to these conversations, we can shape them as they evolve.

> *"To strengthen your mind, stay informed. Watch the news, understand both sides of situations, have an open mind, and a positive attitude. Read as much as you can. There is no limit to what you can learn."*
>
> *- Heidi Forrest*

Wondering how to CONNECT? Here are ways to get started:

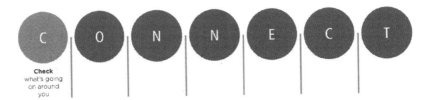

Check what's going on around you

> *"I read business books from visionaries, entrepreneurs. I love to learn. Staying up to date with current events is important as well. News can be negative at times but we should know about the community and environment we live in."*
>
> *- Marika Siewert*

1. **C**heck what's going on around you. The world moves fast, and so should you. Keep yourself well informed about what's going on in the world and your local community. Find out about major developments in politics, economy, science and health, culture and sports. Having a well-rounded awareness and understanding of these topics is essential, no matter your personal or professional aspirations. Reflect on what each development means to you and those around you. Expect to discuss it with friends and colleagues, at local events or conferences. Pick up the local newspaper, subscribe to reliable and comprehensive publications like *Newsweek*, set up a Twitter

account, sign up for a news feed, or set alerts on your favorite news site to stay on top of new developments.

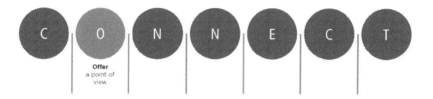

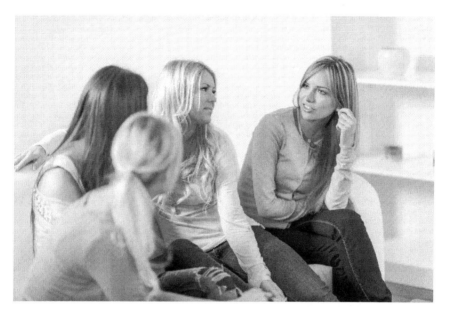

2. **O**ffer a point of view. When we connect, we can't simply be observers or remain impartial. Reflect on the news, interpret the facts and develop an opinion. Join an existing debate—or start a brand-new conversation about a topic you're interested in. You may not always agree, and that's fine. Share your perspectives and viewpoints with others, always in a thoughtful and respectful way.

Some people have an opinion about everything. We all have a family member or annoying colleague who fits that description. Having an opinion about *something* is always a good place to start—ask others for their opinions too. Share something you've learned that you think would be valuable to others. One day you may joke that everyone's entitled to "your" opinion.

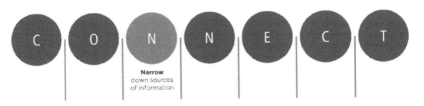

3. **N**arrow down sources of information. Thanks to the internet, millions of sites can publish content that's neither credible nor objective; this kind of information can be misleading and downright false. Just because it's online doesn't mean it's reliable. Even with the reliable sites, it's easy to feel overwhelmed by so many sources to sort through. Be selective about the information you consume. Rely on the most objective and trustworthy sources of information you can find, like the Associated Press, the *New York Times* or the *Wall Street Journal*. These reputable news companies use talented journalists who do their homework to help us navigate through the clutter; they work hard to verify information before releasing it to the public. Think quality, not quantity.

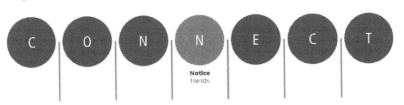

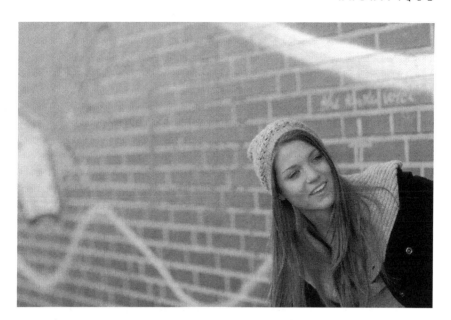

4. **N**otice trends. Assess widespread changes in behaviors, values and opinions, and think about how they might impact your personal or professional goals. Easier said than done? Check out Google Trends (http://www.google.com/trends/), a free tool based on Google Search that reports how often a particular term—"vacation" or "diet," for example—is searched relative to other searches done in a given region or language. You can subscribe to get Trends email alerts for topics you care about. Google Correlate finds search patterns that correspond to real-world trends, such as a recent flu-like illness spreading around that suddenly generated a surge in related searches. The service also presents lists of real-world people, places and things ranked in order of search interest, making it easy to spot new trends.

But Google's not your only resource. "Trending" on Facebook shows you a list of topics and hashtags that have recently spiked in popularity. This list is personalized based on a number of factors, including your location, pages you've liked, and what's trending across Facebook. There are many resources to help you stay connected, keeping an ear to the ground and an eye on what's trending around you.

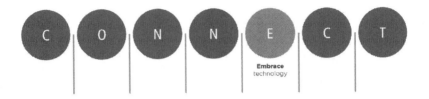

5. Embrace technology. It has changed every aspect of our lives: how we work, how we entertain ourselves, how we conduct our everyday lives, how we consume information and how we connect with each other. It's often referred as the "democratization of information." It's given us all access to an enormous amount of data and helped us stay connected with the click of a button.

    Leverage mobile technology to stay in touch with friends, family members and coworkers. It's so easy these days to check your Facebook feed, message someone or make a Skype or FaceTime video call. Use technology wisely, though: it connects us, but it can also isolate us—as was so brilliantly captured by American rapper and activist Prince Ea in his "Can We Auto-Correct Humanity?" video.

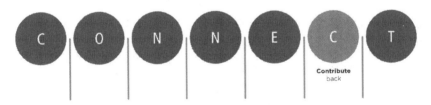

6. Contribute. To really connect, you need to get involved in a personal way. Give back by contributing your resources, time and/or talent to make a difference in other people's lives. Join a non-profit. Help out at a local church or volunteer at a community center. Find ways to use your gifts to help others and make a difference. When you contribute to your community, you make a more profound connection that helps you understand and appreciate your own environment more deeply.

*"It's every person's responsibil-
ity to tap into his or her network
of fans and to leverage connections
for good causes and non-profits."*

- Melanie Kannokada

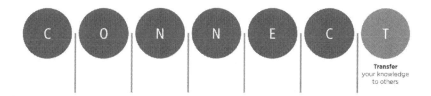

Transfer
your knowledge
to others

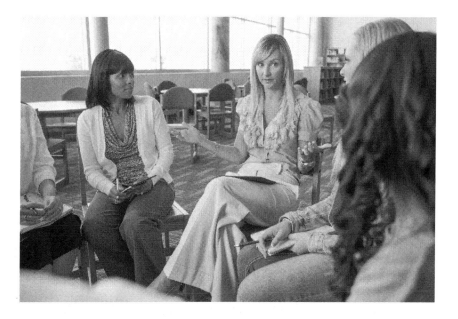

7. **T**ransfer your knowledge to others. Share what you learn. You may run into an insightful article, catchy post, funny picture, or a stunning video that touched you or inspired you. Tell your friends, family, coworkers, and your followers or fans why it moved you or what you learned from it. Spread meaningful ideas.

If you're a singer-songwriter like former *American Idol* phenomenon Kelly Clarkson, use your musical gifts to share messages that inspire. Clarkson has a personal connection to the songs she picks, and she wants to share her knowledge with others: "I think I gravitate toward songs with a defiant message because I always feel like I'm fighting just to be me." Her songs often focus on messages of independence and self-empowerment for women.

Clarkson's story is certainly one of defiance. Her parents divorced when she was six, and her mother struggled financially while raising the children. Clarkson worked small jobs as a telemarketer and a cocktail waitress. When she appeared on the first season of *American Idol,* her apartment had recently burned down and she was struggling financially.

> "*The times that I have felt the most beautiful were times when I was doing something to help other people, and was living a healthy life style. People don't get involved in enough positive ways in their community.*"
>
> *- Heidi Forrest*

Despite her incredible success as an artist, Clarkson has never lost sight of her past, and she continues to share it with others. Today, she's an international music icon selling millions of albums and topping billboards around the world with titles like "Breakaway" and "All I Ever Wanted." Someone once said, "Gaining knowledge is the first step to wisdom. Sharing it is the first step to humanity." We are truly human when we connect with others.

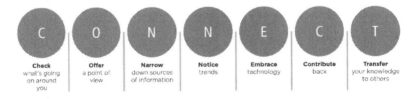

Check	Offer	Narrow	Notice	Embrace	Contribute	Transfer
what's going on around you	a point of view	down sources of information	trends	technology	back	your knowledge to others

MASTER

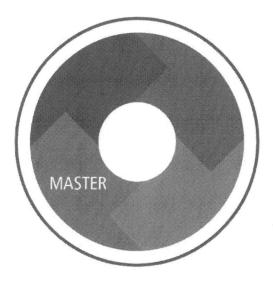

Effective communication is key to achieving results on a personal and business level. Developing and mastering verbal and written communication skills is essential. Our ability to express our thoughts and ideas concisely—with simplicity, clarity, conviction and eloquence—allows us to impact and influence others. As Jacqueline Kennedy Onassis said, "Once you can express yourself, you can tell the world what you want from it."

Many studies have shown that strong writing and presentation skills promote access, opportunity, professional achievement and future success. Conversely, weak communication skills create major roadblocks to success in many facets of life. If we confuse others, we weaken our argument, we look unprepared and unprofessional, and others see us as having less credibility and value. Good communication skills improve our interactions with others, building stronger relationships based on mutual understanding.

> *"It's not always what you say, but how you say it that matters."*
>
> *- Kristen Dalton*

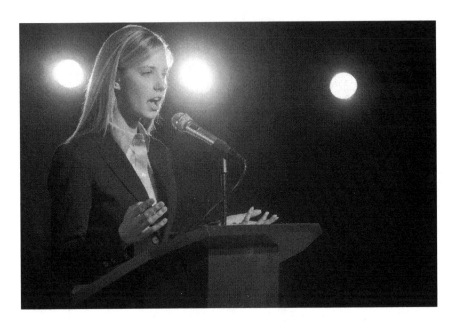

In the past few decades, the need for skillful written and verbal communication has accelerated with the use of email, word processing and presentation software. You may have to prepare presentations for meetings, send recap emails and status reports to team members, or write a proposal for senior management. No matter your job or profession, you're likely to communicate with colleagues through a mix of written, oral and non-verbal (body language, facial expressions) means as you explain, negotiate, persuade, motivate and inform. This requires interacting with people in an efficient and appropriate manner to deliver information quickly and clearly, avoiding misunderstanding and confusion.

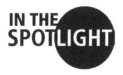

IN THE SPOTLIGHT

Toastmasters International Tips for Public Speaking

Toastmasters International is a non-profit organization that teaches public speaking and leadership skills. It published the following tips based on years of best practices by its members:

1. **Know your material.** Pick a topic you're interested in. Know more about it than you include in your speech. Use humor, personal stories and conversational language–that way you won't easily forget what to say.

2. **Practice. Practice. Practice!** Rehearse out loud with all equipment you plan on using. Revise as necessary. Work to control filler words. Practice, pause and breathe. Practice with a timer and allow time for the unexpected.

3. **Know the audience.** Greet some of the audience members as they arrive. It's easier to speak to a group of friends than to strangers.

4. **Know the room.** Arrive early, walk around the speaking area and practice using the microphone and any visual aids.

5. **Relax.** Begin by addressing the audience. It buys you time and calms your nerves. Pause, smile and count to three before saying anything. ("One one-thousand, two one-thousand, three one-thousand." Pause. Begin.) Transform nervous energy into enthusiasm.

6. **Visualize yourself giving your speech.** Imagine yourself speaking, your voice loud, clear and confident. Visualize the audience clapping–it will boost your confidence.

7. **Realize that people want you to succeed.** Audiences want you to be interesting, stimulating, informative and entertaining. They're rooting for you.

8. **Don't apologize for any nervousness or problem** – the audience probably never noticed it.

9. **Concentrate on the message**–not the medium. Move your attention away from your own anxieties and focus on your message and your audience.

10. **Gain experience.** Mainly, your speech should represent you—as an authority and as a person. Experience builds confidence, which is the key to effective speaking. A Toastmasters club can provide the experience you need in a safe and friendly environment.

Source: Courtesy of Toastmasters International

It's vital to learn basic principles of effective communication and apply them daily to real-life scenarios. Employers want employees who are strong communicators, whether they're presenting to others or writing clear email messages. How do you become a MASTER communicator?

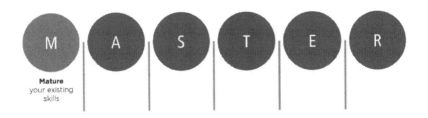

Mature
your existing
skills

1. **M**ature your existing communication skills. We're all born with basic communication skills so we can function and grow. We learn a few more things along the way, at school, at work and in social settings. We also tend to forget what we learned, or take these important skills for granted. We're always in learning mode. Take a refresher class on business or creative writing to learn ways to get your points across in clear, concise and compelling language. "What's the point of my communication? What's my narrative? Should I use multimedia? What's a catchy title? How much content is too much—or not enough? When can I use humor?" These are among the most important things you'll ever learn to accomplish your business objectives and extend your influence.

> *"I had the opportunity to learn valuable communication skills including public speaking skills. It's not something you are born with. You have to work at it. I wouldn't be the person I am today if I did anything differently in my life.*
>
> *- Connor Boss*

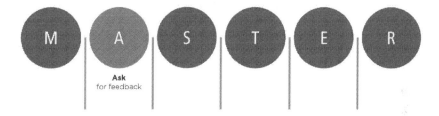

Ask
for feedback

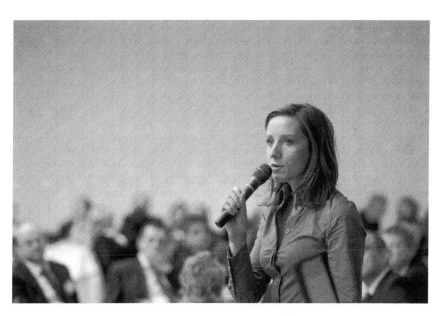

2. **A**sk for feedback. It's very challenging to assess our own communication skills. If you've ever rehearsed a speech watching yourself in the mirror or taping yourself, you know what I'm talking about. We all need help to evaluate how we communicate with others. Invite a friend, family member, coach, mentor or colleague to review and

critique your written or oral content and presentation. Do you have a clear agenda and objectives? A compelling setup? A concise delivery? A strong message? An engaging style? Are you using the right language for your audience? Should you use more visuals or shorter sentences? It takes courage to ask for feedback, and to actually take it in. Be brave: ask for advice on how to improve the quality and effectiveness of your communication.

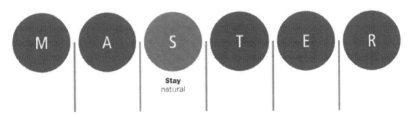

3. **S**tay natural. Don't force it. Be authentic. What you say and how you say it must be genuine or you'll lose your audience. Make it an enjoyable experience for others and yourself. You're more likely to get your message across, engage your audience and get the results you're looking for if you act naturally. Easier said than done, though.

> "A friend of mine once told me, 'I wish someone told me that when you get to the top, there is nothing there.'"
>
> - Marika Siewert

Ask English singer-songwriter sensation and Grammy Award winner Adele. Staying relaxed and natural when facing a large crowd is challenging even for her:

I get so nervous on stage I can't help but talk. I try. I try telling my brain: stop sending words to the mouth. But I get nervous and turn into my grandma. Behind the eyes it's pure fear. I find it difficult to believe I'm going to be able to deliver.

Yet to her millions of fans, Adele looks completely natural and authentic on stage. How else would anyone successfully "Set Fire to the Rain"?

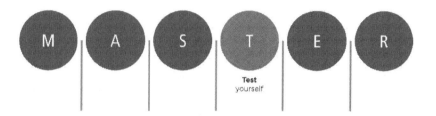

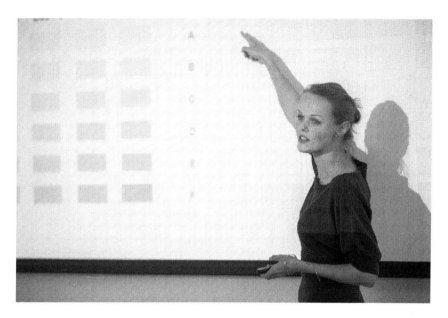

4. **T**est yourself. There's no better way to know how well you're prepared than by courageously practicing what you learned in the real world. If you haven't already done so, you may be hesitant. Speaking in front of a crowd is known to be one of the scariest things some people will ever do. Join a local Toastmasters chapter (http://www.toastmasters.org/) to develop and test your presentation skills. Seize any public speaking opportunity in your professional or social life. You'll build confidence over time. Explore what works and what doesn't—and adjust accordingly. Commit to learning through ongoing testing and experimentation: it's the only real pathway to mastery and excellence.

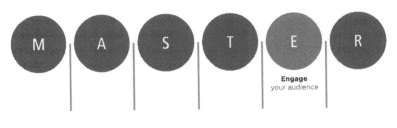

Engage
your audience

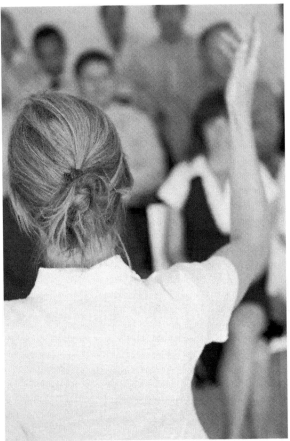

5. **E**ngage your audience. To connect with them, you must address them in a way that's deeply relevant. Know their sensitivities and triggers. Understand what matters to them, and adapt your content and approach accordingly. Ask questions. Seek participation from them. Anticipate objections like "Why should I care?" and "What's in it for

me?"—questions commonly faced by those who fail to understand and engage their audience.

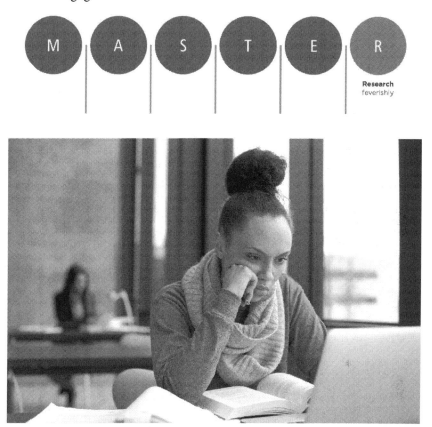

Research
feverishly

6. **R**esearch feverishly. You can only achieve mastery through complete dedication, continuous improvement and research. Research what works and what doesn't. Research new techniques. Pick up one of the countless books or access some of the infinite online resources focused on strengthening communication skills. Watch quality videos like conference keynotes or TED Talks that offer brilliant storytelling-style presentations on every possible topic. Learn from them: refine your communication style and content by studying others and researching constantly.

> *"Be prepared. Preparation is crucial to any endeavor in life. You start by conducting a self-assessment. What are your thoughts or beliefs on hot button topics? Ask yourself why you feel this way about it. Do your research, then provide a thoughtful point of view and deliver in a diplomatic way."*
>
> *- Kristen Dalton*

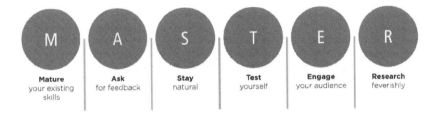

M	A	S	T	E	R
Mature your existing skills	**Ask** for feedback	**Stay** natural	**Test** yourself	**Engage** your audience	**Research** feverishly

Consider the following recommendations by one of the nation's top communication experts, and you'll soon be ready to truly MASTER how you communicate with others.

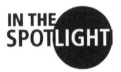

Top Seven Recommendations by Communication Expert Robyn Hatcher:

1. Know your communication style (something I call your ActorType) and identify its strengths and weaknesses. No two people are alike, so the communication style of one person may not be effective for another. Learn to polish and emphasize your communication strengths, and minimize and reframe your weaknesses. You can take my ActorType quiz at http://www.speaketc.com/.

2. Stand with confidence. It can take as little as two seconds to make a first impression, and 60-80% of that first impression is nonverbal. So it's important to use confident body language. Standing: make sure your feet are hip-distance apart, weight slightly forward & evenly distributed on both feet; don't cover your torso by folding your arms or standing behind a podium.

3. Watch your tone. The tone and inflection of your voice is the second most important part of your communication (right behind the visual). Habits like "up-speaking" (making everything sound like a question), "drop-speaking" (losing energy at the end of the sentence, and "whatevering" (using a boring singsong rhythm) weaken your message and make you sound less confident.

4. Choose your words wisely. Choose words with power, impact and imagery. Use metaphors & analogies to appeal to the right brain and help people visualize what you're saying. Lose non-words like "like," "um," and "you know"—words that minimize you and your message. Words like "little," "maybe," "just," "I think," "kind of" and "sort of" make you sound unsure, weak and less-than-confident.

5. Remember WIIFT (What's in it for Them.) People take action based on logic and emotion. Emotional reasons often have the most impact. When you're trying to engage your listener, try to connect to an emotional need your listener may have; think about what you have to *give* them, and not just what you *need from* them.

6. Define your bottom line. Within an hour, people forget 40% of what you say. Before you present or engage in an important conversation, think about the one thing you want the listener to remember. Then build your presentation or conversation around that bottom line, using logical & emotional support. Repeat the bottom line at least three times if possible and appropriate.

7. Communicate your greatness. What are the specific core character strengths and experiences that set you apart from your peers? Don't be shy about sharing them. I believe we all have incredible talents and greatness inside, and it's our duty to share them. Not confident about your strengths? Share them anyway. The act of sharing them will make you more confident. People suggest "faking it till you make it"—but nobody likes a fake. So I prefer to say: "Own it while you hone it." Or "Act like it's a fact."

Follow the principles we reviewed in this chapter (and summarized below) and you'll be well underway to unleashing the potential of a stronger, more effective mind.

Listen	Learn	Connect	Master
Let others know that you are listening	Look up information	Check what's going on around you	Mature your existing skills
Identify the right environment	Embark on a new learning opportunity	Offer a point of view	Ask for feedback
Seek clarification	Acknowledge you don't know	Narrow down sources of information	Stay natural
Think without judging	Reach out to your network	Notice trends	Test yourself
Engage with eye contact	Navigate your way through failure	Embrace technology	Engage your audience
Notice non-verbal cues		Contribute back	Research feverishly
		Transfer your knowledge to others	

Although all four practices (Listen–Learn–Connect-Master) are crucial to strengthening our mind's abilities, we also value them differently depending on our individual needs and competencies. For example, I discovered that most women value, or at least associate these principles with, a strong mind in this order: learning from successes and mistakes (Learn), staying well informed (Connect), listening well (Listen) and finally, mastering verbal and written communication (Master).

IN YOUR OPINION, WHAT CONTRIBUTES TO A STRONG MIND?

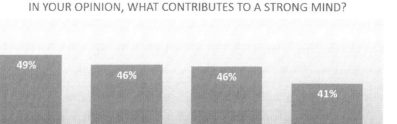

49%	46%	46%	41%
Learning from successes/mistakes	Staying well informed (news)	Listening well	Mastering verbal/written communication

If you meet Sara Blakely, founder of the Spanx company and one of the 100 most influential people in the world according to *TIME* magazine, you'll soon realize that she not only listens well, learns quickly and connects brilliantly—she's also a master at communication. By applying the "Mind Journey Wheel of Success" principles, you too can accomplish wonders and tap into the amazing potential of your beautiful, open mind.

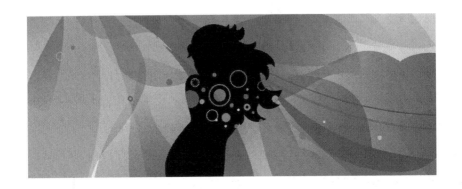

"Character contributes to beauty.
It fortifies a woman as her youth fades.
A mode of conduct, a standard of courage,
discipline, fortitude, and integrity
can do a great deal
to make a woman beautiful."

- Jacqueline Bisset,
English actress,
Golden Globe and Emmy Award nominee

CHAPTER SIX

BECOMING CONFIDENTLY BEAUTIFUL

If you ever wore a "silver leotard, leg warmers, and a shiny headband" in an aerobics class, you know that it takes more than a tiny bit of confidence. Raised by an ophthalmologist father and a mother with a PhD who worked as a French teacher, this young woman understood the value of a good education. At the top of her class in high school, she went to Harvard University; then-economics Professor Larry Summers became her mentor and thesis advisor. After graduation she enrolled at Harvard Business School and earned an MBA with highest distinction. When Summers became Treasury Secretary in 1999, he asked her to join him in Washington DC as his Chief of Staff; she was only 29 years old. Inspired by technology's potential to transform people's lives, she moved to Silicon Valley to pursue a dream.

This talented woman is Sheryl Sandberg; her name now symbolizes confidence and success for new generations of equally ambitious women. Sandberg joined Google in 2001 as Vice President of Global Online Sales and Operations. A few years later she was hired by then-23-year-old Facebook founder Mark Zuckerberg as Chief Operating Officer; she ran business functions including sales, marketing, business development, human resources, public policy and communications. In the first three years of her tenure as COO, Facebook grew to an astonishing 800 million users, with $2 billion in annual revenue.

Sandberg is considered one of the most influential people in the world and a source of inspiration to millions of women. This accomplished executive has a remarkable track record. Amid her job responsibilities at Facebook, the mother of two wrote a book for professional women that landed on top of bestseller lists the day it launched. *Lean In: Women Work and the Will to Lead* encourages women to "lean in" to positions of leadership and not "lean back" when it comes to their personal and business lives. With unprecedented influence, Sandberg inspired an international movement among professional women looking for ways to support each other and deal with roadblocks to their professional ambitions.

Now one of the youngest female billionaires in the world, Sandberg is a role model for women seeking work-life balance. Her astonishing success was only possible by combining talent and vision, a razor-sharp business acumen, an ability to listen, communicate authentically and inspire others—and perhaps most importantly, self-confidence.

Every time you update your status or check your newsfeed on Facebook, take a second to reflect on what Sandberg has accomplished. In *Lean In* she asks women, "What Would You Do if You Weren't Afraid?" The question is inspiring, and lies at the core of a fundamental challenge faced by countless women in our society: low self-esteem and lack of confidence that prevent them from pursuing their dreams. But a confident, assertive woman can move mountains and accomplish wonders with sheer determination and conviction.

> *"Confidence is something you build. In anything I do in life, I spend a great deal of time researching, researching and researching. Know what you want to do. The better prepared you are, the more likely you are to meet that goal."*
>
> *- Susie Castillo*

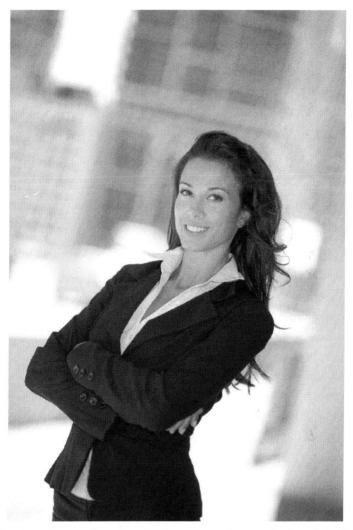

Now imagine confronting similar personal or professional challenges, but also going through life with a serious speech impediment, or hearing or vision problems. Many inspiring stories of women with disabilities have illustrated the importance of emotional strength and confidence in getting ready for life's challenges. Lizzy Velasquez is a remarkable woman who inspires many through her courage, strength and confidence. A successful motivational speaker and author, Velasquez has a rare medical condition that prevents her body from storing fat and building muscle: as a result she has zero percent body fat, never weighs more than 64 pounds, and has a weak immune system and visual impairment. Her unusual physical appearance led to a life of endless stares—she was once labeled the "World's Ugliest Woman" on YouTube. But despite these challenges Velasquez never let her physical appearance—or online bullies—define her. Her positive attitude has been nothing short of contagious.

> *"The number one challenge for women today is that we all compete and compare. No matter how accomplished you are, there will always be someone ahead of you. So don't define yourself by your appearance or accolades. Everyone is on a different journey: do the best with where you are right now and own it. A confident woman is a beautiful one."*
>
> *- Kristen Dalton*

These inspiring examples, whether in the business world or in everyday life, show us that being confidently beautiful is the surest path to personal success and happiness. We immediately recognize poise and self-assurance when we meet someone who gives us a firm handshake, makes direct eye contact, uses a lower vocal tone and a calm voice.

What is confidence? Are some of us predisposed towards it? Can we really be confident if we lack self-esteem? Do women and men express confidence in the same way? So many questions, yet there are so few answers—"confidence" is not a common subject of study in school. Research has shown that risk taking, failure and perseverance are essential to confidence building. We're confident when we believe in certain principles and are ready to defend them no matter what. When we act decisively, trusting our own judgment and not letting others interfere. When we're certain that our chosen course of action is the right one. When we exhibit determination without being aggressive.

Confidence is gained through personal life experiences. It involves four skills that I outline below; these essential skills will help you strengthen your self-confidence in what I call the "Confidence Journey Wheel of Success":

- **INSPIRE:** Influencing and inspiring others
- **ADAPT:** Embracing change and overcoming ambiguity
- **LEAD:** Leading by example and driving toward outcomes
- **AFFIRM:** Strengthening through failure and the power of conviction

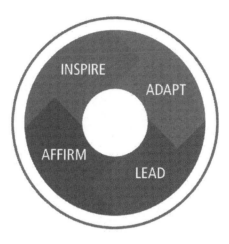

Figure 1 Confidence Journey Wheel of Success

INSPIRE

How well do you know yourself? "Who am I?" is the most difficult question for many of us to answer—yet it's the most powerful way to boost confidence. According to Greek philosopher Aristotle, "Knowing yourself is the beginning of wisdom."

Think about how you want to see yourself. Knowing yourself gives you wisdom and strength. When you know yourself, you're less likely to be influenced by other people's perceptions, and *more* likely to influence and inspire others. You're strong when you can speak with confidence about yourself, your identity, your dreams and aspirations.

Have you ever wanted to know what it would be like to enter a room and command attention? To have others compelled to listen? We're confident when we know where we came from, where we're going, what we want, how to pursue our goals and avoid distractions. We're grounded, confident and inspiring when we truly know ourselves, care for others, share our own experiences, show our vulnerabilities, identify with others and influence how they think. Consider Malala, the Pakistani schoolgirl who survived an assassination attempt by the Taliban and who *Newsweek* called "the bravest girl in the world." She influenced and inspired millions around the world to stand up for their beliefs and let their voices be heard.

Here are some essential ways you can INSPIRE others:

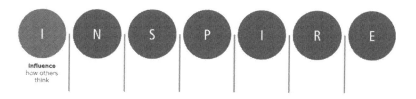

1. **I**nfluence how others think. Those who are gifted at convincing others use no voodoo magic or superhero powers. Instead they exhibit a strong sense of self, show deep respect, sensitivity and compassion. They read situations and people well, and have a burning desire to win people over to their way of thinking. They communicate their ideas assertively, but in a way that values and respects others.

When we inspire others, they're eager to hear our thoughts and ideas. When we challenge traditional ideas or offer new ways of thinking, we offer them new perspectives that expand their horizons. We influence how people see the world and encourage them to think outside the box.

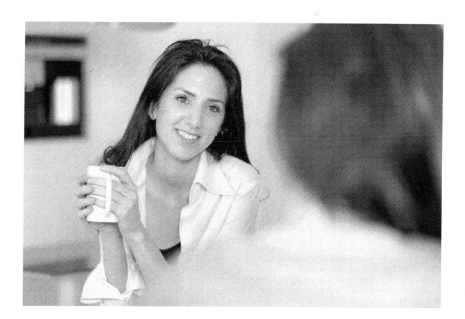

It's not surprising that Robert Cialdini's *Influence: The Psychology of Persuasion* and Dale Carnegie's *How to Win Friends and Influence People* are considered some of the best self-help books ever published. Cialdini introduced six ethical principles of influence (reciprocity, scarcity, liking, authority, social proof and commitment/consistency) that are critical dimensions of effective human interaction backed by social-scientific testing. Among Carnegie's twelve recommendations on ways to win people over—many of them inspired from fundamental sales and marketing techniques—he argued that we can best influence people when we honestly try to see things from their point of view, tackle a challenge and appeal to nobler motives. Although experts differ on the most effective ways of influencing others, they all agree that these common-sense principles from psychology can be learned and applied to everyday situations.

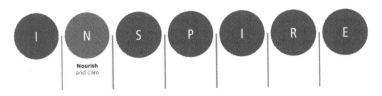

2. **N**ourish and care. Caring for others (without an expectation of receiving anything in return) is arguably one of the purest forms of motivation and inspiration. Generosity can take many shapes: sharing knowledge or skills, giving time or resources. Those who care, and who show they care by their actions, inspire us: they make us feel important, sing our praises, give encouragement and moral support when it's most needed, and share their wisdom and expertise. We don't question their motives. They build trust and goodwill; their generosity brings out the best in individuals, organizations and communities. They inspire us to do our part, to return the favor and give to others.

> *"Don't get distracted. Be purposeful in everything you do. Set realistic goals and pursue them. And take time for friends and family. Value them. They keep you grounded in good and bad times."*
>
> *- Marika Siewert*

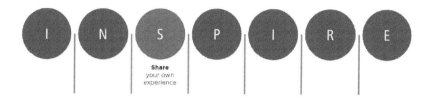

3.   **S**hare your own experience. Personal stories captivate us and capture our hearts. We listen better when people share their own personal stories with us because we can relate to their life experiences, fears, struggles, aspirations and hopes. Every story is worth telling—so is yours.

This explains the popularity of the "Experience Project" (www.experienceproject.com/), a site offering the world's largest collection of life experiences, thoughts and personal stories organized by theme (travel, family, health, hobbies, relationships and more) or popularity. Inspire others by opening up and sharing your own experience with them. Tell them what you learned and how it changed you. You'll be glad you did—and you may learn a thing or two about yourself in the process.

> *"Few people know that I battled homelessness during my senior year of high school, and had to live separately from my family. Success is triumphantly overcoming obstacles that have potential to stop you, and having the courage to carry on through life altering circumstances. Because you are one of 7 billion people on earth doesn't mean that you can't make a difference. You just need the willpower and the passion."*
>
> *- Heidi Forrest*

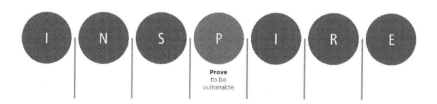

4. **P**rove to be vulnerable. Our culture has conditioned us to think about vulnerability as a weakness instead of a strength. Most of us fear vulnerability. In a brilliant and funny TED Talk called "The Power of Vulnerability," social work professor Brené Brown explores why we struggle with vulnerability—and more importantly, why we shouldn't numb ourselves to it. Brown, who spent the past ten years studying courage, compassion, authenticity and shame, says that the answer lies in embracing our own vulnerability and imperfections: "to let ourselves be seen, deeply seen, vulnerably seen; to love with our whole hearts, even though there's no guarantee." She urges us to "recognize that we are enough."

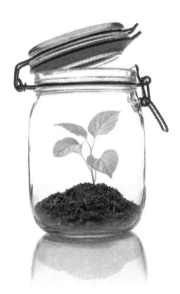

When we let ourselves be vulnerable, something remarkable can happen. Diagnosed with metastasized papillary thyroid cancer at age 12, with extensive tumors that spread to her lungs, Esther Earl had a hard time breathing. Despite a worsening illness that kept her from experiencing a normal teenage life, Earl injected her sense of humor and empathy into the social media world, blogging and posting videos that made her a YouTube sensation. She became friends with author John Green, inspiring him to write the worldwide bestselling book and Hollywood hit *The Fault*

in Our Stars. Earl lost her battle with cancer shortly after she turned 16. Her parents founded This Star Won't Go Out, a non-profit organization to help families who have a child with cancer. To this day, Earl remains a brilliant example of the transformative power of vulnerability and courage, no matter our individual circumstances.

> *"You have to love yourself, know who you are, learn and grow from experiences to succeed in life."*
>
> - *Connor Boss*

Uncertainty and risks are part of existence. By showing ourselves to be vulnerable, by exposing who we really are and how we feel, we connect in ways that wouldn't otherwise be possible. When we meet someone who is comfortable with herself, who doesn't attempt to hide her fears and weaknesses, we're inspired.

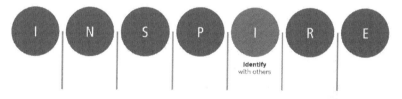

Identify
with others

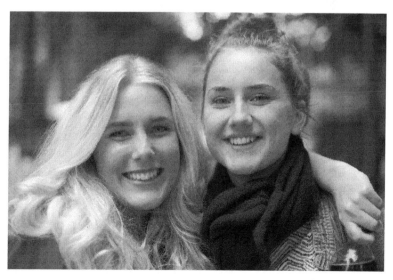

5. **I**dentify with others. Our ability to connect with others, wholly or partially, draws us closer and builds a sense of emotional attachment. When we talk in terms of another person's interests, when we genuinely care about them and show it, we inspire them. Empathy allows us to recognize emotions in others. Be understanding of someone else's ideas, feelings and interests. Take a genuine interest. Be considerate and compassionate and you'll inspire them.

Lara Logan, one of the world's best foreign war correspondents, dedicated her life to reporting from battlefields in war zones from Egypt to Afghanistan to Iraq. Often embedded with the American Armed Forces, she has influenced our understanding of events unfolding in all corners of the world. She helped us identify with others far away from home. Logan, who has been the chief foreign affairs correspondent for CBS News since 2006 and a correspondent for CBS's *60 Minutes,* has inspired millions of women through her courage and dedication to award-winning reporting from war zones, often putting her own life at risk. While covering the Egyptian Revolution celebrations for *60 Minutes,* her crew was handcuffed at gunpoint; she was beaten and sexually assaulted by a mob in Tahrir Square. She broke the silence a few months later by speaking out about sexual violence against women, especially female journalists in war zones. In Logan's case, her reporting serves a greater agenda of compassion, awareness and understanding.

> *"When you have a high value of self, you can give so much more to others. You can move with confidence. That is called beautiful."*
>
> *- Maureen Francisco*

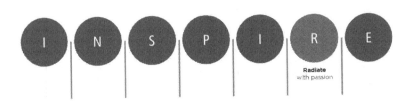

Radiate
with passion

6. **R**adiate with passion. All charismatic individuals have a gift that sets them apart from everyone else. This gift has two elements: a deeply rooted, resilient sense of purpose, and a profound passion that's both inspiring and contagious. Their passion is so strong, so absolute, we can't help but want to find and pursue our own dreams with equal intensity and devotion. Passionate people inspire us.

No one radiates greater passion and conviction than British actress, screenwriter and author Emma Thompson. The two-time Academy and Golden Globe Best Actress award-winner is well known for a stellar career featuring performances in *Howard's End*, *The Remains of the Day*, *Harry Potter* and the recent *Saving Mr. Banks*. Thompson is perhaps less known for her dedication to important causes: she's an ambassador for the charity ActionAid and a supporter of Greenpeace, Elton John AIDS Foundation and the Refugee Council. She's also President of The Helen Bamber Foundation, a human rights charity based in London that provides therapeutic care, medical consultation, legal protection and practical support to survivors of human rights violations.

> *"Devote yourself to helping others*
> *and success will follow: well-being,*
> *happiness, and self-esteem."*
>
> *- Heidi Forrest*

I was fortunate enough to meet Thompson in London while assisting her and portrait photographer Nick Haddow in their efforts to raise awareness about human rights violations and sex trafficking. Having witnessed first-hand her amazing commitment to helping others over the years, I can truly say that the word "passion" reflects her footprint and her legacy.

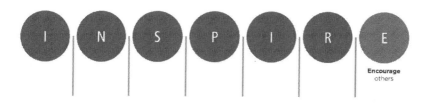

Encourage
others

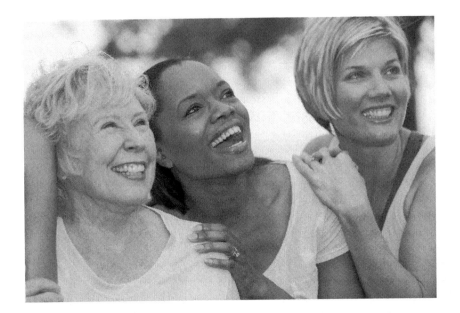

7. Encourage others. Everyone needs encouragement at times. Remind them that they made the right choices, that they needn't be discouraged when progress takes longer than planned, that they can be patient and persevere no matter the roadblocks or setbacks. We inspire when we support others and comfort them.

Named one of the "Most Influential People in the World" by *TIME* magazine in 2012, Kate Middleton—the Duchess of Cambridge, wife of Prince William—is the perfect example of someone who knows how to encourage others. Aside from her widely publicized fashion sense, the Duchess has found inspirational ways to support and encourage others. She's an active and committed supporter of children's hospices that provide vital lifelines to children and families affected by life-threatening conditions and need a caring, fun place to call home. Her royal activities, charitable patronages and speeches have fostered greater awareness and support for this cause, and have provided much-needed encouragement for the children and those who care for them. Her Royal Highness The

Duchess of Cambridge, Countess of Strathearn and Lady Carrickfergus is *magnifique* inside and out.

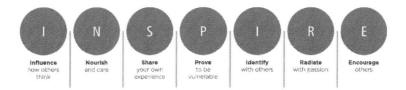

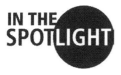

She Is Malala

If confidence had a face, it would be that of a young Pakistani school-girl who became a symbol of bravery and hope for women around the world by her 16th birthday. Her name is Malala Yousafzai, and her story is like none other.

Malala is outspoken in a world where speaking out can cost your life. The daughter of an educational activist, Malala refused to be silenced. She had been vocal about educational rights in a region where the Taliban had banned girls from attending school. She started blogging for the BBC under a pseudonym at age 11, writing at length about the life of a young woman under Taliban rule. After her words were picked up by newspapers and television channels, the Taliban saw Malala's defiance and confidence as a threat to their authority in the region. One afternoon, she boarded her school bus like any other day. But on that day, October 9, 2012, a Taliban gunman entered the bus and shot Malala in the head. The shot nearly killed her. She was 15 years old. In critical condition for days after this heinous and cowardly crime, she miraculously survived.

Malala's courage and confidence became a powerful source of inspiration. She received massive worldwide media coverage and outpourings of support from millions, including politicians and celebrities from U.S. President Barack Obama to Madonna to Angelina Jolie. Malala touched the heart and soul of anyone who values equal rights and the right to education, and anyone who admires those courageous enough to face adversity and ignorance no matter the consequence or price.

Malala was featured on *TIME* magazine's front cover as one of the "The 100 Most Influential People in the World." She received the Nobel Peace Prize along with many other national and international awards, including the National Youth Peace Prize and the Ambassador of Conscience Award from Amnesty International. Her book *I am Malala* became a bestseller and a powerful testimonial for generations of women. Malala is an extraordinary young woman who showed us that confidence is beautiful and can serve more than a personal agenda: it can inspire women around the world to stand up for their beliefs.

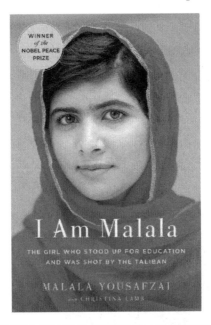

ADAPT

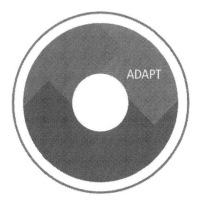

The ability to adapt is particularly important in today's world of constant change. Change can be intimidating: we may not want to challenge the status quo because things have always been done a certain way—or simply because we're too comfortable. We use expressions like "that's the way we've always done it" and "don't fix what's isn't broken." But resisting change means looking back instead of forward. We can't grow or get anywhere in life if we always fear change.

Change is to the human condition what oxygen is to the environment. Our ability to adapt as humans has kept us alive for centuries. As individuals, leaders and community members, we must not only embrace change—we must drive it! We must challenge ourselves, get out of our comfort zones, learn (or re-learn) and be open to new ways of doing things.

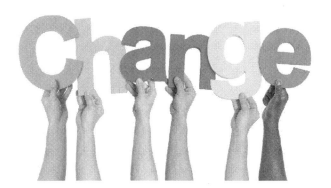

> *"Don't take life too seriously. Things can change in seconds. You can be greatly success-ful one minute and not the next. Enjoy the journey and have fun along the way. Find the right balance between work and a social life."*
>
> *- Brittany Dawn Brannon*

We live in a world where uncertainty is the only certainty. Yet most of us want to avoid the ambiguity that comes with change. We seek clarity. We demand transparency. We wish for simplicity. We expect life to follow certain patterns and we fear the unknown. But we can't escape it: our work responsibilities can be unclear after a reorganization or after someone leaves. Our relationship status can be uncertain after a fight or a separation. Our financial future can be unpredictable after we lose a job or make the wrong investments. In this environment, confident people don't get set back. They don't get paralyzed or destabilized by the unknown. They know what must be done: they stay focused. They move forward in confidence. Others look up to them. They light the path for others to follow. They know where they're going, even in the darkest moments.

> *"I had a lot of rejections in my life. I wanted to go to my dream school, Stanford. I was waitlisted at first. If I didn't fight for it, it would have never happened. Things didn't come easy to me. It only motivated me to work hard at everything I did, so no one could deny me the opportunities I wanted to pursue."*
>
> *- Melanie Kannokada*

What does it take to ADAPT?

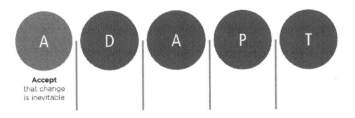

Accept that change is inevitable

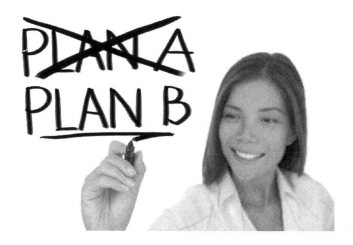

1. Accept that change is inevitable. Change is the only constant these days. New ways of doing our jobs, new skills to build, new colleagues, new neighbors—and the list goes on. Technology has contributed to this fast-changing environment where it's not "if" but "when" change will take place. Have your plan B ready.

    Learn to see change as a good thing. I mean "change with a purpose," not just "change for the sake of change." Change is vital: those who can adapt are simply more successful than those who won't or can't. English naturalist and geologist Charles Darwin put it brilliantly:

    it is not the most intellectual of the species that survives; it is not the strongest that survives; but the species that survives is the one that is able best to adapt and adjust to the changing environment in which it finds itself.

> *"No matter how much money you make, be true to yourself. Failure keeps you alive. Stay grounded at all times."*
>
> *- Brittany Dawn Brannon*

Accept change: let it unfold.

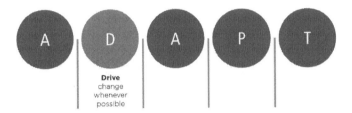

Drive
change
whenever
possible

2. **D**rive change whenever possible. When we accept the notion that change is part of everything we do, our perspective alters. We're no longer caught by surprise, struggling to keep up with it. We step back and seek to understand the origin of a change, its trajectory and how it contributes to reaching our goals. We consider what's next and how to push forward. We feel empowered. We dream big.

Once we accept change with a healthy dose of enthusiasm and confidence, we actually run towards it: we welcome a new world of possibilities. We no longer wait for it, we're no longer a victim of it—we become the *source* of positive change. We actively contribute to change because we firmly believe it will alter our future (and the future of others) for the better. To drive change, we must have a purpose and a destination in mind. Motion without progress is wasteful. The change must come from a solid place: knowing what it will bring and how it will contribute to a better world.

> *"I built my confidence over time. I had a poor image of myself at first. I lost weight, carried myself a different way. Ultimately, I stood up and felt great about myself. It's not something you are born with. You have to work at it."*
>
> *- Connor Boss*

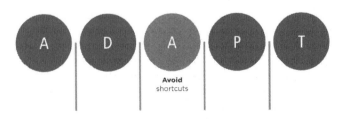

Avoid
shortcuts

3. **A**void shortcuts. Everyone's in a hurry these days. We speed-date, text and tweet when we shouldn't, grab fast food on the way home, look for six-week-miracle nutrition or exercise programs. We take shortcuts in almost every facet of our lives. Shortcuts save us time, money and effort—all things we never seem to have enough of. But shortcuts are often too good to be true, and we over-estimate what they can do for us. We also don't think about the consequences, the side effects we may not see right away. We learn the hard way and pay the price.

> *"Whether you go on a date, an inter-view or a meeting at a record label company... you show up! You decide how much respect you get."*
>
> *- Marika Siewert*

Don't take shortcuts unless you know the upside is far greater than the potential downside. Take the time to breathe and consider your options before acting. Don't take shortcuts that erode your confidence and self-esteem. To adapt to rapid change, avoid the temptation to get there quickly and at all costs.

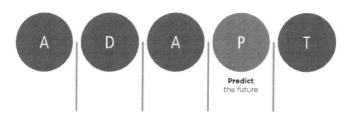

Predict
the future

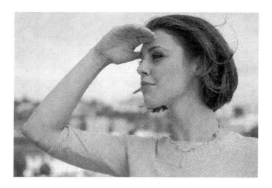

4. **P**redict the future. A source of fascination for centuries, the ability to predict the future has been a topic of research and a source of literature in recent history too. A four-year study organized as part of a government-sponsored forecasting tournament called the "Good Judgment Project" (goodjudgmentproject.com) proves that a small group of participants are "super forecasters." These skilled individuals, coming from all walks of life, can far more accurately predict the probability of an event than other participants—they're even better than intelligence officers who have access to classified information. These "super forecasters" are open-minded people, critical thinkers who consistently see problems from all sides and embrace uncertainty.

> *"I wouldn't be the person I am today if I did anything differently in my life. I am happy with the choices I have made."*
>
> *- Connor Boss*

Rest assured, though. You don't need to be a "super forecaster" to be confident and predict the future. We're not talking about predicting the future of the world, but rather your own. Some people believe that past actions can help us predict future behavior and events. It often can, as history tends to repeat itself. But only to a point. Confident people have a vision for the future—one that may involve a different course than the past might have suggested. As Abraham Lincoln said, "The best way to predict your future is to create it."

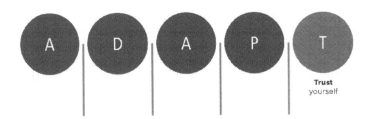

Trust
yourself

5. **T**rust yourself. You can adapt and welcome even light-speed change if you trust yourself to be ready for it. Trusting yourself is about

having self-awareness (knowing who you are) and self-confidence (knowing what you can do). We tend to build trust when we have success, but we can't build success without failure. Failing is an important development process. It's essential to learning what works and what doesn't, and to applying these lessons to our jobs and personal lives. Trust is earned. It's built over time. Trust yourself and discover your amazing ability to adapt.

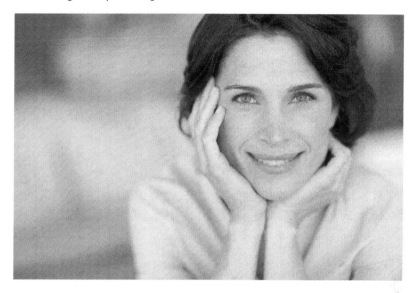

Self-confidence is no foreign concept to 1st Lt. Melissa Stockwell, a U.S. war veteran and Bronze Star and Purple Heart recipient. Stockwell, an above-the-knee amputee, is also a Paralympian and paratriathlete. In 2004, Lieutenant Stockwell's life changed forever. At the age of 24, she lost her leg when a roadside bomb exploded during a convoy in Baghdad. She received a prosthetic leg 52 days after losing her real one; in her eyes, she was one of the lucky ones. Stockwell trusted herself and pushed her limits, accomplishing feats that most of us can't even imagine. She became the record holder for the 100-meter butterfly and the 100-meter freestyle in the 2008 Paralympic Games. Moving on to compete in paratriathlons, she was named USAT Paratriathlete of the Year in both 2010 and 2011. The three-time Paratriathlon World Champion is now a triathlon coach and a motivational speaker. Don't tell Stockwell what she can or can't do—she knows better.

"Don't listen to people who don't know who you are or pretend that they do. More importantly, learn quickly to put up with criticism. You will real-ize that it is a critical skill set."

- Brittany Dawn Brannon

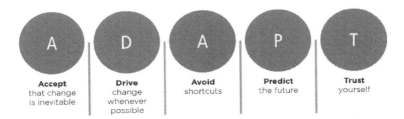

Accept
that change
is inevitable

Drive
change
whenever
possible

Avoid
shortcuts

Predict
the future

Trust
yourself

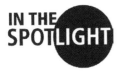

IN THE
SPOTLIGHT

You Can't Eat Beauty!

"You can't eat beauty! It doesn't feed you" are words all-too-familiar to academy award-winning actress Lupita Nyong'o. This is what her mother repeated to her growing up. In her moving, heartfelt "Black Women in Hollywood" acceptance speech where she admitted strug-gling with low self-esteem in her youth, Nyong'o added, *"Those words bothered me; I didn't really understand them until finally I realized that beauty was not something I could acquire or consume. It was something that I just had to be."* Nyong'o opened her emotional speech by recount-ing a letter she received from a young black girl who, so inspired by the actress's success story as a talented black woman, decided not to buy skin-whitening cream.

Born in Mexico City, raised in Kenya until the age of sixteen, Nyong'o returned to Mexico to add Spanish to the list of other languages she speaks (English, Swahili and Luo). She continued her education in the U.S., completing a master's degree in acting from the Yale School of Drama. She earned numerous awards and nominations, including the Academy Award for Best Supporting Actress for her role in Steve McQueen's drama *12 Years a Slave*.

Today, Nyong'o is so much more than a rising Hollywood star or the new face of Lancôme. In her acceptance speech at the seventh annual Black Women in Hollywood Luncheon, she shared a remarkable perspective on what beauty stands for: *"What is fundamentally beautiful is compassion for yourself and for those around you."* She concluded so brilliantly with, *"There is no shade in that beauty."*

LEAD

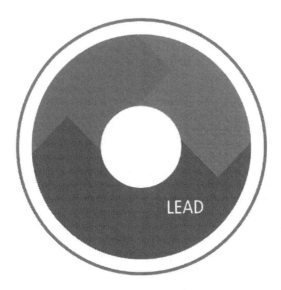

"Do as I say, not as I do." We've all heard this expression. We've all received advice from people willing to dispense it but unwilling to show us the right way. They may say one thing and do quite another.

Leading by example is easy to say but hard to do. It's also one of the most meaningful ways to show true character and integrity. When we lead by example our words, actions, beliefs and values are all in alignment. We walk the talk. This is the true signature of a leader and role model.

We're all busy driving our personal and professional agendas. How we do so varies significantly. Some of us are more action-oriented than others. When we have clear goals and organize our days around specific results, we tend to be more effective. We focus our time and energy on things that matter most. We are results-oriented: we know where we're going and why, and we make things happen. We demonstrate a tremendous sense of confidence to others.

"Find your strength. Don't look at other women and compare yourself to them in order to define who you are. Know yourself by looking inside."

- Connor Boss

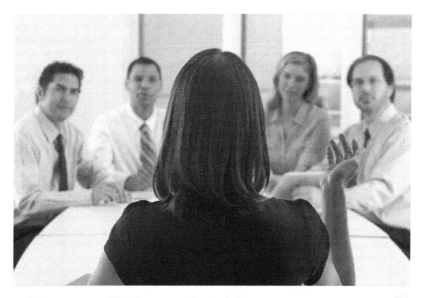

How can you LEAD most effectively?

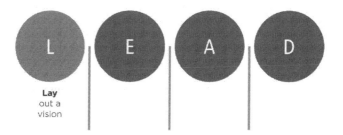

Lay
out a
vision

1. **L**ay out a vision. Effective leaders provide a clear picture of the future, and suggest a path to reach it. Others want to follow in their footsteps as they embrace that vision and seek to be part of it. A vision without a plan is short-lived, though. It might intrigue, but it won't succeed in moving others in that direction. Without vision, an individual or an organization won't know where it's going or how to get there.

To lay out a vision, you need a clear purpose and equally clear values and beliefs. If we have a vision for our future, we can make things happen. With a vision, we can move mountains. We can transform the world. In business, it requires an ability to recognize new opportunities and trends around us, anticipate threats and roadblocks before they appear, and develop a strategic company direction. But laying out a vision goes far beyond the business world. Confident women can articulate a vision for themselves, their family or the community they serve, and create a plan to see it through.

> *"I would advise any woman to start with having a clear goal. Then you can decide how much you want to put into meeting that goal. For me, it's about doing what it takes to get to the end goal."*
>
> *- Connor Boss*

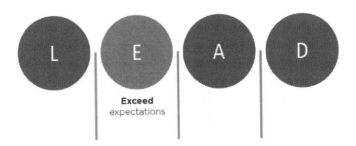

Exceed
expectations

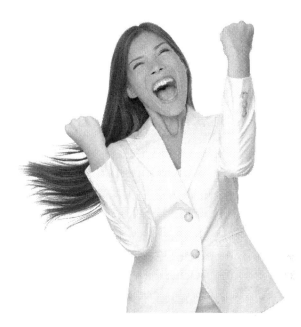

2. Exceed expectations. Under-promising and over-delivering is a rare leadership quality, but it's crucial to building trust and inspiring others. I've seen this quality valued more than gold in the business world. Failing to meet expectations is considered unacceptable. Exceeding expectations is the ability to go the extra mile, to go above and beyond, and to demonstrate absolute commitment to excellence.

We want to be over-achievers and encourage individual or team excellence, but at the same time we're careful not to build a culture of perfection where failure is not an option. Instead, let's find genuine ways to better manage expectations so they're realistic and let us deliver more. We're not talking about sand-bagging objectives or lowering the bar, but about giving ourselves room to surprise and delight others.

> *"I don't need to live anyone else's life because I get to be the leading lady in my own incredible story."*
>
> *- Marika Siewert*

If anyone knows about exceeding expectations, it's Gabrielle Reece—otherwise known as "Gabby." A pro athlete and a Women's Beach Volleyball League star, fitness icon, model and writer, Gabby has left few stones unturned in her life. Once named "One of the Five Most Beautiful Women in the World" by *Elle* and one of the "20 Most Influential Women in Sports" by *Women's Sports & Fitness*, Reece is Nike's first female athlete to design a shoe, and the company's first-ever female cross-training spokesperson. She's now a popular contributor on wellness, health and fitness, with articles appearing in magazines like *Shape* and *Elle,* and a writer for Yahoo Health, *The Huffington Post* and the *Los Angeles Times Magazine.*

> *"If you are pretty on the surface and if that's it, then you are not really beautiful. But inner truth, knowing one's self-worth, being proud of who you are, impacting people positively, that's really beauty in my eyes."*
>
> *- Melanie Kannokada*

An avid proponent of empowering people to take responsibility for their own health, Reece has developed a range of functional training workout kits and DVDs specifically for women. The mother of two has also written two popular books—*Big Girl in the Middle* and *My Foot Is Too Big for the Glass Slipper: A Guide to the Less Than Perfect Life.* Reece is a source of inspiration for many. She has never ceased to exceed expectations—at least ours.

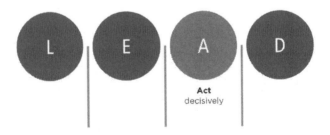

L E A D

Act
decisively

3. **A**ct decisively. Effective decision making is the very essence of leadership; it's a skill that simply must be acquired and mastered. Everyone wants to make good decisions: to accept the right job, buy the best car, surround ourselves with the right people. No matter the decision, if we fear failure, procrastinate or take too long gathering information in making a decision, we simply miss out altogether on opportunities.

Acting decisively requires courage, determination, accountability and a drive to take action. You don't want to make decisions rashly either, without carefully assessing the situation, evaluating options and anticipating consequences. Make them deliberately and within a reasonable timeframe. We admire those who can make tough decisions, decisively. We're also inspired by those who hold themselves fully accountable to the decisions they make.

> *"I quickly learned that I will survive if I*
> *am able to get out of my comfort zone.*
> *Every time I am faced with an uncomfort-*
> *able situation, I embrace that challenge."*
>
> *- Maureen Francisco*

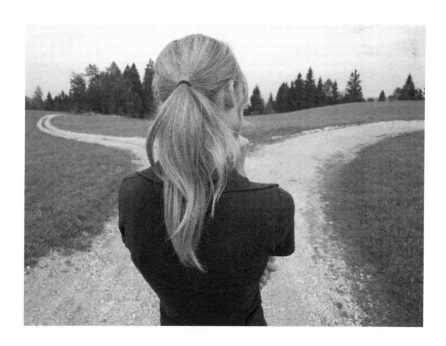

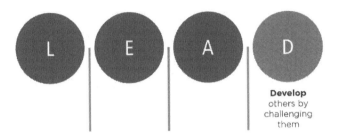

Develop
others by
challenging
them

4. **D**evelop others by challenging them. Most of us had coaches, teachers or parents who pushed us to do more, go faster or work smarter. No matter the challenge, they expected more from us. We learned to expect more from ourselves, which opened new doors and changed our perspectives. They challenged us to stretch our limits and to fully realize our potential.

Coaching champion and master motivator Pat Summitt holds the most all-time wins for a coach in NCAA basketball history. One of the most successful women's basketball coaches in the nation with eight NCAA basketball titles, she's the only coach in NCAA history (one of three college coaches overall) with more than a thousand victories. She knows a thing or two about developing others.

> *"Get involved with your community. It helps to have people's support and to support others."*
>
> *- Heidi Forrest*

Summitt's coaching approach has been about challenging players:

In my 38 years as head coach of the Tennessee Lady Vols I have preached the following things: absolute dedication, unselfishness, unwillingness to give up, determination to see every contest to the very end.

In 2011, Summitt met a new and very determined opponent: early-onset Alzheimer's. Her approach was consistent with her coaching style, declaring, "Put away your hankies. There's not going to be any pity party. We're going to fight, and we're going to fight publicly."

Summitt is considered one of the greatest and most inspiring coaches of all time for many reasons. Among them is what she often said about coaching players: "they don't care how much you know, until they know how much you care." This is so amazingly true.

Apply the following recommendations by confidence expert Christine Serb and LEAD by example.

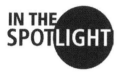

IN THE SPOTLIGHT

Top Seven Recommendations by Confidence Expert Christine Serb:

1. **Get to know your potential.** "The biggest obstacle in life between you and your goal is you." Where are you on your potential grid? Your potential is dependent on your actions. Step out of your comfort zone. You can be a 10 out of 10 if you work on your abilities. How do you do that?
    a. Learn about your abilities. Find something you can do particularly well and work even harder at it.
    b. Don't make excuses—everyone does. Make *efforts*.
    c. Let others see your full potential at work. Be proud.

2. **Follow your purpose with passion.** It's amazing how confident you'll feel when you're living your passion. Passion is doing what you were destined to do.
    a. Follow the fire that burns within you.
    b. Keep a laser focus on the desired outcome. Take one step at a time. Following your purpose is a journey.
    c. Look for the few things that make the most difference.

---

3. **Think positive, stay energized.** "Train your mind to see good in every situation." Your passion will energize you. Life can be difficult, conflict will arise, pressure will challenge you, but your passion will keep you energized.

    a. Remember: You're the master of your destiny. Thoughts are very powerful—what you say to yourself, you become.

    b. Cut out negative people in your life.

    c. Rethink challenges. Consider how things are possible rather than impossible.

4. **Listen to your inner wisdom.** "If you listen to what you know instinctively, it will always lead you down the right path." It's not what we know, but what we *decide*. Rise up and stand for what your inner voice is saying.

    a. Follow through with every intuition you have.

    b. Follow thorough until you see something all the way to completion.

    c. Always follow your instincts.

5. **Take risks and learn. Do not fear to fail.** "If you're not willing to fail, you're not willing to succeed." Negativity is not to be ignored—it's to be *conquered*.

    a. Determine what's holding you back, and choose to face your fears.

    b. Decide what's important to focus on—be prepared.

    c. Focus on your outcome; let your success propel you.

6. **Be assertive in your communication.** "It's not what you say, it's how you say it." Assertive people command respect because they know what they want.

    a. Discern what is and what is not within your control.

    b. Stay away from words like "have to," "should," "need" and "can't." Don't say "sorry!" for no reason.

    c. Ask clarifying questions when you disagree with someone, rather than going along with it.

7. **Adopt a winning attitude.** "Life is 90% attitude; the other 10% is what happens to us." Thinking positive is internal, but having a winning attitude is external.
   a. Take responsibility to challenge yourself regularly.
   b. Tell yourself, "if is to be, it's up to me."
   c. Your mind is like a garden: what you plant on the inside will show up on the outside. A winning attitude is a mindset.

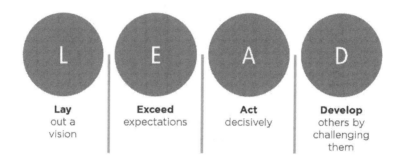

Lay
out a
vision

Exceed
expectations

Act
decisively

Develop
others by
challenging
them

AFFIRM

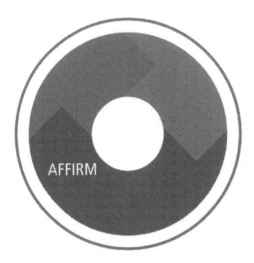

In every mistake lies an opportunity for personal growth. Mistakes are stepping-stones to learning, whether we learn from our own mistakes or those of others. As Thomas A. Edison put it, "I have not failed. I've just found 10,000 ways that won't work." Learning from our mistakes means we won't repeat them. It also means that we affirm our commitment to perseverance and self-improvement. If we learn from mistakes, shouldn't we hope to make more—not fewer—in the pursuit of wisdom?

Confidence comes from our ability to face the world without fear. One of the greatest mistakes anyone can make is being too afraid to make them.

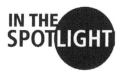

IN THE SPOTLIGHT

The Confidence Gap

Is lack of confidence the reason so many women are still missing out on opportunities in the corporate world? Is confidence more important than competence? We all know competent individuals who lack confidence; the reverse can be harder to detect. It's no surprise that success has more to do with confidence than it does with competence.

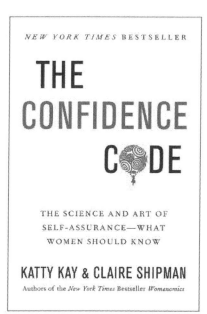

In *The Confidence Code,* journalists Katty Kay and Claire Shipman look for answers in genetics, neuroscience and psychology to understand why women struggle with confidence, and why they limit their career opportunities based on feelings of self-doubt. This problem apparently impacts women of all ages, and at all stages of their career. Why do women under-estimate their abilities or their performance? Why are they so demanding of themselves? By seeking perfection they often feel they fall short of their own expectations, an issue of self-perception more than anything else.

Kay and Shipman interviewed women leaders from the worlds of politics, sport and business, trying to understand why overqualified, well-prepared women are still holding back from pursuing amazing opportunities. Their male counterparts are often less knowledgeable, less qualified or less capable, but they come across as more self-assured, a trait that rewards those who exhibit it. Studies have shown that women don't initiate salary negotiations or get the same outcomes as men. What can women do about it?

Kay and Shipman explain that, despite the fact that confidence is largely influenced by genetics, it's within our reach to think positively, take risks and become confident. They suggest that becoming less people-pleasing, less perfectionistic, and *more* willing to take action and risks are the key ingredients to filling in the confidence gap.

How can you learn to AFFIRM? Here are some places to start.

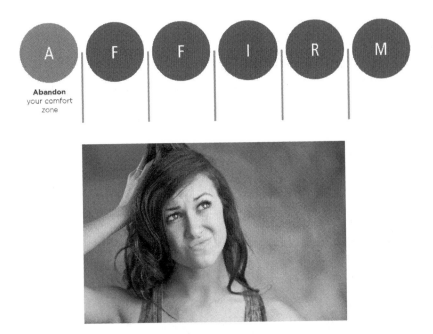

A — **Abandon** your comfort zone

F

F

I

R

M

1. **A**bandon your comfort zone. Things that make life worthwhile and bring out the best in us lie outside our comfort zone. Find your comfort zone—that warm, cozy, stress-free, safe place—so you know where it is . . . and then stay far away from it!

   Risk-taking is what defines great leaders who step out of their comfort zone (no matter how awkward or difficult that is), push themselves and test their limits. The sacrifice, effort and diligence required to push our limits is far greater than some are willing to commit to. They nestle into their comfort zone, not realizing it's limiting their potential. So do something you've never done before. Do something that scares you—and do it before your security blanket suffocates your adventurous spirit!

   > "Some women have lost faith and do not believe they are beautiful. Past relationships, family situations, betrayals, negative words may have contributed to the way they feel. Yet these things are not real. We are all born unique, with a purpose and different skills and talents to offer the world. We must focus on our strengths. Remember that you are more than enough and you are worthy."
   >
   > - Kristen Dalton

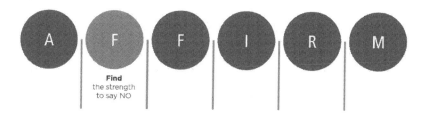

2. **F**ind the strength to say "NO!" Despite what you may have been told at school, the most difficult word in our vocabulary isn't "pneumonoultramicroscopicsilicovolcanokoniosis"—the longest word in any of the major English language dictionaries (it refers to a lung disease). The most difficult word is actually the shortest: a simple, undeniably clear "no."

Why is it so hard to say no? Why don't we say it more often? We're conditioned to believe that saying no hurts, or takes greater effort and energy. When we use it, we feel guilty and that we have to explain ourselves. We don't want to disappoint and we don't want to be judged—no matter the consequences. We over-commit—and ultimately fail those we're trying so hard to please.

We say yes because we haven't set healthy barriers in our relationships with others. But by learning to say no to others, we effectively learn to say yes to ourselves. Once we're confident enough to say it, we experience a renewed sense of freedom and control. By saying no, we can focus on what really matters to us. No need to go into lengthy explanations—and no hard feelings either. The confident individual can say no firmly and respectfully; as a result, she can build a reputation that serves her personally and professionally. When you say no, there's no need to apologize either. In the video "Not Sorry," the hair care brand Pantene urges women to stop apologizing, act with confidence and conviction, and to "shine strong."

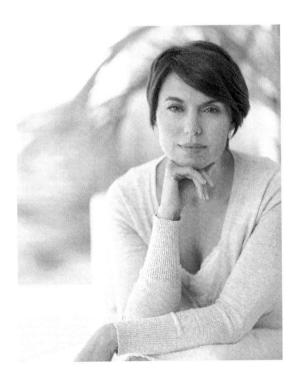

"My album is called "Unstoppable" because I am."

- Marika Siewert

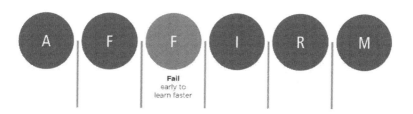

Fail
early to
learn faster

3. **F**ail early to learn faster. By now, we've established that failing is necessary to learning. But failing early on is preferable, since we can apply what we learn earlier in our lives. It takes a tough skin to be a risk-taker in the early part of our career or personal life. We certainly have less to lose, but we may not be adequately mature or prepared for gleaning valuable lessons from failure. We owe it to ourselves to try anyway.

> *"I love learning. I love testing my capabilities. I always look for new opportunities to be the best I can be in every field I approach and apply myself where I can have most impact."*
>
> *- Melanie Kannokada*

Unfortunately, schools often promote different skill sets, and the pursuit of perfection gets in the way of taking chances. If there's little margin for error, why would we risk it all by pushing ourselves into unknown territory? This way of thinking is a major roadblock to creativity and innovation, two important skill sets that require repeated experimentation, trial and error. Being confident means embracing learning through failure as early as possible—it puts us a step ahead of everyone else.

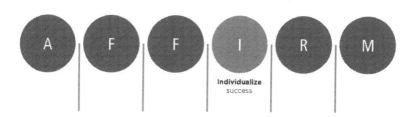

Individualize
success

4. **I**ndividualize success. Success is quite personal, really. We define our own criteria and set our own targets. When we don't, we let others define what success looks like, along with how successful we are in their eyes.

We also need to own our own approach to living a successful life and the principles we follow. It's not uncommon to be inspired by our religious community's principles, our culture's values or our family's ethics. We're the sum of these many parts—but we ultimately create our *own* blueprints for work and life success. Don't let anyone else create them for you.

Bethany Hamilton has her own personal way of defining success. In 2003, at the age of 13, she was attacked by a 14-foot tiger shark while surfing off Kauai's North Shore. The attack severed her left arm just below the shoulder. After losing over 60% of her blood and undergoing multiple surgeries, Hamilton was still determined to pursue her dream of becoming a professional surfer. Despite the trauma, she returned to the water on a surfboard less than a month after the incident.

According to Hamilton, her faith is her backbone. It has profoundly shaped her approach to life, giving her hope and strength when she most needed it. Just over a year after the shark attack, she won the Explorer Women's division of the 2005 NSSA National Championships; she later turned pro. Hamilton's story of perseverance and determination has been the source of much media interest; she shared her story on *The Today Show The Ellen DeGeneres Show* and more. Her story eventually was turned into a major motion picture, *Soul Surfer.*

> *"I learned about what character means. When my name wasn't called out as the winner, I didn't let that experience paralyze me from finding my next success. If you don't overcome it, life starts happening to you as opposed to you doing something with your life."*
>
> *- Maureen Francisco*

Consider the following recommendations by the country's top Chief Inspiration Officer to assert yourself as a true leader and individualize your idea of success.

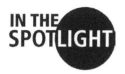
IN THE
SPOTLIGHT

Top Seven Recommendations by Chief Inspiration Officer Bobby Bakshi (www.ResonantInsights.com):

1. **Be clear about who you are.** You are in integrity when the life you're living on the outside matches who you are on the inside. You are in integrity when your thoughts, words and action are congruent. Only you know when you are being true to yourself. Get clear about how *you* define your integrity, not based on what the external world might think.

2. **Listen to your anger.** All our emotions teach us more about what's most important to us. Suppressed emotions— particularly anger— are toxic to our body and mind. Misdirected anger typically has grave consequences. Anger is an opening to more deeply knowing yourself. Typically, underneath anger is fear. Under fear is grief. And under grief is a return to joy—our natural state of being. Feel your emotions; get curious about what triggers them. That awareness leads to making choices that are congruent with your inner truth and your integrity.

3. **Shine light on your shadows.** To paraphrase Carl Jung, our shadows are those things we hide, suppress or deny. We all have shadow stories. Most of us have secrets we've never shared, or shared very selectively. We grow when we learn why we choose to keep secrets. We grow even more when we can release them honestly: first with ourselves and then with those we love. Shed light on your shadow and learn deeper truths about your inner beauty.

4. **Know your fear and own your power.** Often we hold secrets because we're afraid: of what people will say, of not being good enough. Regardless of whether you share your shadows/secrets with others, acknowledging to yourself what you're afraid of is the beginning of greater freedom and owning your own power.

5. **Forgive, for yourself.** Most life stories that start with anger about someone else typically circle back to us. The sooner you forgive others, the sooner you get out of the victim consciousness. In her book *Left to Tell*, Immacuée Ilibagiza shares her miraculous story of how she survived the Rwanda genocide in 1994: she and seven other women huddled silently together in the cramped bathroom of a local pastor's house for 91 days! Ilibagiza shows us how to discover the power of forgiveness, truly unconditional love and understanding—through our darkest hours.

6. **Be you—everyone else is taken.** Take a day (or a week!) to assess all your choices: what you wear, how you interact with people, and so on. At the end of each day, honestly assess whether your actions were 100% your choice or based on subconscious beliefs about what you "should" do. Drop choices that aren't in integrity with your true self.

7. **Discover and live your purpose.** Once you're clear about who you are, and accept yourself just as you are, you can confidently articulate and live your personal values and purpose. Purposeful lives are not reserved for the Mother Teresas of history. There is no big or small purpose. Living your unique gifts fully is why you're here. Don't shy away from shining your light and being all you can be. Now, go be all you're here to be!

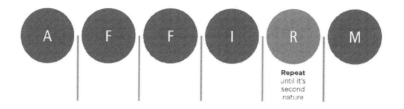

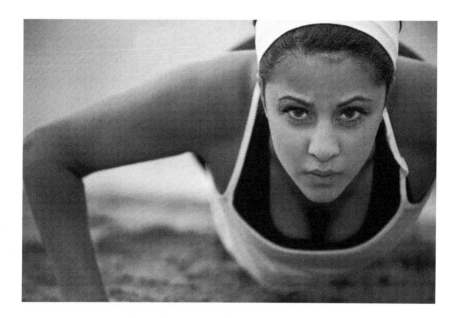

5. **R**epeat, repeat, repeat. Repeat your practice again and again until you get so skilled that it becomes second nature. We often use the old adage, "practice makes perfect." Science has shown that it's true: after extensive practice, our brain's working memory kicks in. We master new skills and find our "zone" where our actions become coordinated and fluid. It's true in arts and entertainment, politics, sports and business. When we practice repeatedly, we minimize errors and frustrations over time. No matter your profession or the skill set needed to reach your goals, practice over and over again until your performance is no longer part of your conscious state. When you master a skill, you can perform it with absolute confidence and control.

> *"We all make excuses. Instead, I believe in myself. I set positive goals, practice and persevere until I am completely successful."*
>
> *- Heidi Forrest*

No one knows better than Dara Torres that practice is essential to success. The world record-holder and Olympic swimming medalist has had an amazing career. Growing up in California, Torres began practicing at an early age. She set her first national record at age 12. Her athletic accomplishments (she competed in five Olympic Games) are nothing short of remarkable. Torres has proven that even when you reach the top of your game, you can always improve your skills. Her book, *Age Is Just a Number: Achieve Your Dreams at Any Stage in Your Life,* speaks volumes about her competitive spirit and dedication to self-improvement.

During the Olympic Games in Beijing, Torres set an American record and was also recognized as the oldest Olympic swimmer in the games' history. At age 40, just over a year after giving birth to her first child, Torres won the 100-meter freestyle at the U.S. Nationals; three days later she beat her own 50-meter freestyle record, set 26 years before. Although she fell short of making the 2012 Olympics swim team at age 45, her determination, self-discipline and dedication to practice allowed her to win twelve Olympic medals during her long career.

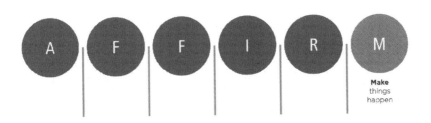

A F F I R M

Make
things
happen

6. **M**ake things happen. Actions speak louder than words. People inspire us when they make things happen. Confidence is a belief in your ability to overcome obstacles—a belief that stimulates decision and action. Conversely, low confidence leads to inaction. When individuals

hesitate because they aren't sure, they hold themselves back. Action is a clear mark of confidence. Confident individuals are resourceful and committed; they find ways to make the impossible possible. They earn a reputation for turning ideas into actions. They're not just observers—they're doers who seize the moment and unleash skills and resources to build, launch, implement, manage and deliver. They act. They want to be known or remembered for their actions.

> *"I want my children to understand*
> *that they can change the world.*
> *We must all lead by example."*
>
> *- Marika Siewert*

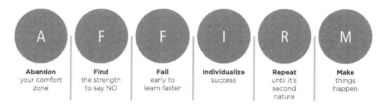

| **Abandon** | **Find** | **Fail** | **Individualize** | **Repeat** | **Make** |
| your comfort zone | the strength to say NO | early to learn faster | success | until it's second nature | things happen |

The principles we reviewed in this chapter are all within your reach. Follow them and you'll soon feel—and become—confidently beautiful.

Inspire
- [ ] Influence how others think
- [ ] Nourish and care
- [ ] Share your own experience
- [ ] Prove to be vulnerable
- [ ] Identify with others
- [ ] Radiate with passion
- [ ] Encourage others

Adapt
- [ ] Accept that change is inevitable
- [ ] Drive change whenever possible
- [ ] Avoid short-cuts
- [ ] Predict the future
- [ ] Trust yourself

Lead
- [ ] Lay out a vision
- [ ] Exceed expectations
- [ ] Act decisively
- [ ] Develop others by challenging them

Affirm
- [ ] Abandon your comfort zone
- [ ] Find the strength to say NO
- [ ] Fail early to learn faster
- [ ] Individualize success
- [ ] Repeat until it's second nature
- [ ] Make things happen

Although all four practices (Inspire–Adapt–Lead–Affirm) are vital to building self-confidence, as in prior chapters, we value them differently based on our individual goals. I discovered that most women associate self-confidence with influencing and inspiring (Inspire), leading by example, being action oriented (Lead), embracing change (Adapt) followed by showing conviction (Affirm). There's no right or wrong answer as to the ideal balance between these four key practices. They're all important in their own ways, and complement each other.

IN YOUR OPINION, WHAT CONTRIBUTES TO SELF-CONFIDENCE?

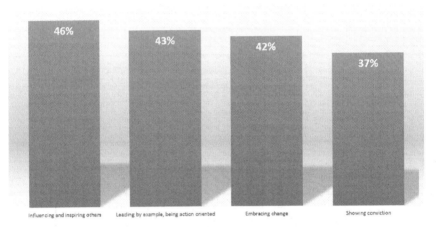

| Influencing and inspiring others | Leading by example, being action oriented | Embracing change | Showing conviction |

We All Walk in Different Shoes

Meet Aimee Mullins, a gifted athlete, model and actress. She signed a major global contract as a face of L'Oréal, and was appointed a global L'Oréal Ambassador. She was also named one of the world's "50 Most Beautiful People" by *People* magazine. What most people don't know is that Mullins was born with a condition that required the amputation of both legs below the knee when she was only a year old. Despite that challenge, she competed in the Paralympics in 1996 in Atlanta. She set World Records in the 100m, 200m and long jump.

In 1998, Mullins launched her career as a successful model. She modeled for British fashion designer Alexander McQueen by opening his London show on a pair of hand-carved wooden prosthetic legs. She's able to change her height between 5'8" and 6'1" by changing one of her many prosthetic legs. Mullins has been a source of inspiration for many. She has shared her story in countless media outlets around the world, and has become a phenomenon of sorts. She has redefined what it means to make the best out of life and create a true sense of purpose. Mullins embraced momentous change in her life and overcame many challenges along the way. She turned what many of us would consider a severe handicap into a powerful asset that set her apart. She led by example, becoming a change agent and driving positive outcomes for herself and others.

Mullins is a remarkable example of someone who has found strength through adversity and conviction. By following the "Confidence Journey Wheel of Success"—by inspiring, adapting, leading and affirming—you can realize these benefits too. As Mullins says,

> If we want to discover the full potential in our humanity, we need to celebrate those heartbreaking strengths and those glorious disabilities that we all have . . . it is our humanity, and all the potential within it that makes us beautiful.

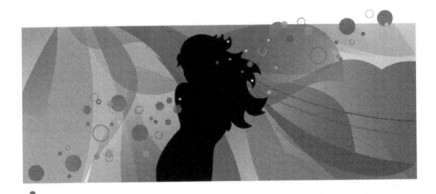

"I know who I am by now.
And I am my own brand."

- Chloe Sevigny,
American actress,
fashion designer and former model

CHAPTER SEVEN

BUILDING THE "YOU" BRAND

Named after a Polish general who helped the U.S. military during the American Revolution, the town of Kosciusko, in rural Mississippi, is an unlikely place to give birth to the most influential brand in the world. Even more amazing are the challenging circumstances a young girl from Kosciusko faced from an early age.

Born into poverty to a teenage single mother, this girl grew up wearing dresses made of potato sacks. Raised by her maternal grandmother until she was six, she was sexually molested starting at nine years old. After running away from home, she became pregnant at age 14, but her baby boy died in infancy. Such a tragic youth would have destined most people to a life of disappointment, suffering and heartbreak worthy of the best talk shows. But this story isn't like any other—and neither is our main character. This is the story of Oprah Gail Winfrey, arguably the most influential woman in the world and the biggest personal brand in recent history.

Named after the biblical character in the Book of Ruth, Oprah's life turned around when she enrolled at Tennessee State University after an oratory contest victory secured her a full scholarship. She earned a degree in speech and performing arts and began co-anchoring the local evening news at the age of 19. Thus began a stellar, fast-paced career in television and entertainment that made her a millionaire at age 32. Today, the "Queen of All Media" is best known for *The Oprah Winfrey Show,* a multiple-award-winning talk show focused on self-improvement and spirituality; her many other roles include TV host, actress, media mogul and producer, to name just a few.

Oprah's story is an inspiring one of personal brand building that created a vast media empire and influenced generations of women. Her brand stands for intelligence, confidence, elegance, credibility, genuine caring and authenticity. These qualities are easy to see in all her work, from her charitable projects like Oprah's Angel Network to her interactions with her talk-show guests. She's believed to be the richest self-made woman in America and the first black woman billionaire in world history; more importantly, she's the most admired woman in the world. Referred to as "The Oprah Effect," her powerful opinions and endorsements of products, books or individuals are instrumental to their success (or failure). "The Oprah Effect" is the ultimate example of personal brand building and how powerful and lucrative a brand can be when managed effectively.

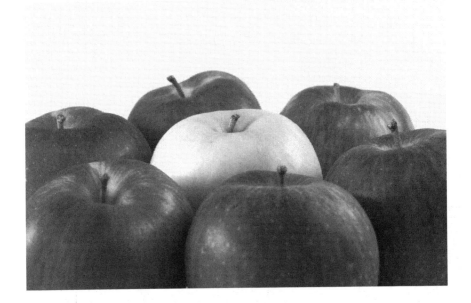

As a marketing wizard by trade, I've always held a deep appreciation for authentic, inspiring brands. Perhaps my real passion is grounded in how brands can make a difference in people's lives. Most people fail to realize how utterly unique they are . . . or they simply fail at communicating that uniqueness to others. Most people never consider how the world sees them or how they want to be seen or remembered. What I'm talking about is the brand identity that makes someone stand out at a job interview, at a meeting with prospective clients, or even on a date with someone special.

> *"Building your image is critical to success in life. Make good decisions about how you appear to the outside world. I personally want to host shows that are classy, that have something to offer to the world and humanity. That's what I stand for. This is part of my identity."*
>
> *- Susie Castillo*

Your brand is the impression you leave on people; it contributes enormously to your success in life. Discovering the real power of personal brands changes your outlook and how you project yourself. Think about what Oprah has accomplished with her astonishing brand identity. Now think about what you can accomplish with yours.

In this chapter, we'll focus on two important topics: *why* you should cultivate your brand, and *how* to begin the process of building it.

It's a Brand's, Brand's World

We live in a culture in which we're constantly bombarded with messages: at work, on the freeway, on email, in social media. Studies have found that the average person receives close to 5,000 messages a day. Many of these messages come from familiar brand names that are part of our everyday lives. Brands are almost companions, expected to make life easier, speed up purchase decisions and deliver better experiences. In some ways, brands are part of us and we are part of them. We all have our favorite brands, whether in fashion, cosmetics, food, drinks or cars.

> *"Most of the issues about beauty and low self-esteem are coming from people not knowing their own identity."*
>
> *- Marika Siewert*

So what makes a brand? To illustrate, I looked at some of the most successful brands in the world and picked one. Let's take a look at Nike, the world's leading innovator in athletic footwear with an easily identified logo and well-known brand values.

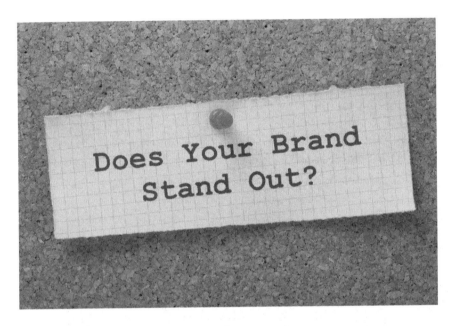

A brand like Nike is essentially the sum of these parts: First, a strong, contagious sense of purpose—one that people can relate to. Nike's mission is to bring inspiration and innovation to every athlete in the world—and according to Nike, if you have a body, you're an athlete! Next, a promise of value showcasing the benefits consumers receive from it. A brand also needs a unique personality with attributes that are one-of-a-kind, relevant and compelling, and that comes to life in people's minds and hearts. Nike's brand personality is known for being exciting, provocative and innovative. A brand provides credibility too, often through success stories and spokespeople. Just as important, a brand fosters an emotional connection with its audience that moves and engages them. Nike's "Find Your Greatness" campaign is an outstanding example here, connecting with us deep down by highlighting the greatness in us all. It touches our hearts with authentic, inspirational stories—and those stories stay with us all the way to the Nike store.

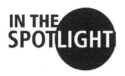
IN THE
SPOTLIGHT

"Find Your Greatness": Nike Ad Campaign

"Greatness is no more unique to us than breathing. We are all capable of it. All of us."

During the 2012 London Olympics, Nike launched one of its most powerful global advertising campaigns, "Find Your Greatness," just as the world focused on the best athletes in the world. The campaign's centerpiece was a film featuring "everyday athletes" that broke through various social media and digital channels. The film, airing on TV in 25 countries, was supported by a global YouTube homepage promotion and Twitter #findgreatness. Athletes were encouraged to share their activities and achievements through social media; their posts were displayed on Nike+ Fuelstream, a dynamic online stream of images and consumer comments. Emotional connection with the videos was immediate—Nike's YouTube channel was flooded with visitors eager to see popular spots like "The Jogger."

Nike's campaign suggests that "greatness" and "achievements" are not "reserved for chosen few." As Nike put it, "It is not just the championship athlete or record breaker that aspires to push their limits. It is also the everyday athlete who strives to excel on their own terms, to set and realize personal goals and achieve their own defining moment of greatness." While the film suggests that each athlete defines their own success, it connects us all through a unifying sense of what greatness can be.

Nike's campaign is a textbook example of effective brand building through emotional connection with an audience, compelling storytelling, and an inspiring, energizing brand message. As the film ends, we're reminded of the "power in seemingly everyday moments from a young boy deliberating a first jump from a high diving board into a pool—a defining moment for him that ends in a final leap into his own moment of greatness." Inspired yet? Clearly, Nike has mastered the art of brand building.

Pick your own brand; think about it in these terms and you'll discover that brands appeal to us from both a rational and an emotional perspective. The same holds true for individuals.

Personal Brand Building

Most people wrongly assume that brand-building techniques only apply to the world of products and services. Though they're inspired by countless years of research and best practices in marketing, brand principles apply to people as well.

> *"I've met so many women who are beautiful in so many ways. They put make up on and go on stage. But how they look has often nothing to do with the woman on the inside."*
>
> *- Heidi Forrest*

Celebrities in business, entertainment, sports and other high-profile careers manage their personal brands as valuable assets that shape their commercial success. Those with a strong brand are far more likely to succeed than those without one. Every sponsorship opportunity they sign up for, every interview they grant, every red carpet event they attend reinforces or weakens their image. Look at actresses like Jennifer Aniston and Angelina Jolie. Both have strong brands that appeal to different audiences, and both make careful choices when representing a brand in a TV or print ad.

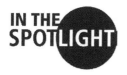
IN THE
SPOTLIGHT

Angelina Jolie and Jennifer Aniston as Brands

Angelina Jolie	Jennifer Aniston
Jolie's top five brand attributes:	Aniston's top five brand attributes:
Seductive	Simple
Sensual	Positive
Mysterious	Personal
Rebellious	Natural
Confident	Approachable
"Femme Fatale"	"Good-Girl-Next-Door"
Product endorsement example: St.John	Product endorsement example: Aveeno

There are no brands more iconic than those of Angelina Jolie and Jennifer Aniston. Both are hugely successful actresses, and both are considered among the most beautiful women in entertainment. Jolie has received an Academy Award, two Screen Actors Guild Awards and three Golden Globe Awards, and was named Hollywood's highest-paid actress for a number of years. She served as Special Envoy and former Goodwill Ambassador for the United Nations High Commissioner for Refugees (UNHCR). Aniston earned an Emmy Award, a Golden Globe Award, and a Screen Actors Guild Award. *Men's Health* magazine voted her the "Sexiest Woman of All Time."

Although the two celebrities have much in common profession-ally (and personally, having both been involved with Brad Pitt), they have distinct brands with vastly different appeal and audiences. This is easy to see in the product endorsements each has pursued. Aniston's "good-girl-next-door" brand identity has landed her opportunities with companies that want to express the "natural," "approachable" nature of products like SmartWater or Aveeno hair products. On the opposite end of the spectrum, Jolie's "femme fatale" brand identity has led her to become the longtime face of upscale American fashion brand St. John., a company that appeals to women in positions of authority.

Are the products endorsed by Jolie and Aniston consistent with their own personal brands? Absolutely. It's clear that personal brands are worth developing and nurturing for celebrities who live in the limelight. But how does that apply to you?

> *"Every woman should know what*
> *her brand stands for. I like to*
> *think about myself as encourag-*
> *ing, positive and inquisitive."*
>
> *- Kristen Dalton*

You don't need to be a Hollywood celebrity or a billionaire entrepreneur to care about your image and your reputation. In fact, you're a brand whether you like it or not. The moment you enter a room or interact with someone, you effectively become a brand. Or, as Amazon.com CEO Jeff Bezos puts it, "Your personal brand is what people say about you when you leave the room." The way you present yourself shapes others' perceptions of you, and determines your ability to pursue your career and personal goals.

> *"Stand up for what you believe in. Know who*
> *you want to be, what you want to be known*
> *for. Be bold. I am a Christian. I often post*
> *inspirational quotes or stories of how God works*
> *in my life. I realize that everyone may not*
> *agree with me and I am at peace with that."*
>
> *- Kristen Dalton*

Your current network of professional contacts—potential employers, business associates and network resources—can easily access your information online, on search engines, Facebook, LinkedIn and more. This is your reputation, available at high-bandwidth internet speed. If you don't manage it to influence how others see or remember you, others will—guaranteed.

Personal branding is the strategy behind the world's most successful people, no matter their profession or their personal ambitions. Brands hold great value—this is why, when faced with two identical products, you're likely to pay more for the one that's branded. The value in your own personal brand will help you accomplish your goals.

Assessing How Others See You

People are complex, multi-dimensional creatures who cannot be defined with a single word or attribute. When describing a friend or family member, we often use multiple adjectives to capture their personality. They're not just "friendly" or "funny" or "smart," but a combination of these traits. People with strong brands are clear about who they are and how they want to be perceived.

> "Know what you stand for and bring this every day into your work or in your charities."
>
> - Brittany Dawn Brannon

Conducting your own brand assessment is essential to understanding how the world perceives you, and creates a basis for your future brand-building efforts.

Here's how it works. You first define your own desired brand attributes: this is the self-assessment step. Second, compare the attributes you chose with what others chose for you: this is others' assessment of you. Third, compare the two assessments and look for potential gaps between them.

There's a myriad of books and online resources to help you conduct your brand assessment, making it much easier to maintain confidentiality of the information you gather from friends, family and co-workers. If you choose to handle the process yourself, print a list of common brand attributes (see the example below) and select the top five attributes that best describe what you want your brand to be.

> *"I am very purposeful with my image. We are in charge of how we are perceived by others. Your brand is whatever you make it. People may see me but may never meet me in person. We only get one chance to make a good impression."*
>
> *- Marika Siewert*

SELECT THE TOP 5 ATTRIBUTES THAT BEST DEFINE YOUR BRAND TODAY

Visionary	Candid	Direct	Dominant	Charming	Humble
Energetic	Traditional	Dynamic	Rigid	Trustworthy	Glamorous
Simple	**Fun**	Confident	Analytical	Free-spirited	Nurturing
Authentic	Aggressive	Straightforward	Decisive	Articulate	Sensitive
Different	Brave	Independent	**Ambitious**	Reliable	Expressive
Agile	Daring	Approachable	Hard-working	Dedicated	Perceptive
Carefree	Competitive	Progressive	Logical	Dependable	**Friendly**
Collaborative	Stubborn	Innovative	Consensus building	Reasonable	Involved
Intelligent	Assertive	Competent	Self-reliant	Nimble	Cooperative
Curious	Driven	Strong	Focused	Adaptable	Open-minded
Original	Resilient	Devoted	Distinctive	Passive	Kind
Intuitive	Sincere	Supportive	Flexible	**Committed**	Poised
Social	Passionate	Gentle	Patient	Helpful	Stylish

Then ask friends, family or co-workers to use the same list and pick five attributes for you (don't let them know what you chose for yourself). Ask them to put their choices in an unmarked envelope so you won't know who said what—people are usually more honest if their input is anonymous.

Next, compile the results in a table (see the example here).

MY SELECTION	NAME 1	NAME 2	NAME 3	NAME 4	NAME 5	NAME 6	TOTALS
Intuitive	Sensitive	Intuitive	Intuitive	Humble	Direct	Kind	2
Fun	Competitive	Fun	Simple	Fun	Original	Fun	3
Ambitious	Decisive	Driven	Driven	Patient	Driven	Dynamic	0
Committed	Committed	Rigid	Committed	Dedicated	Committed	Committed	4
Friendly	Friendly	Reliable	Friendly	Reliable	Reliable	Friendly	3

Here's what will happen. You'll get matches, showing consistency between how you want to be seen and how others see you. Successful individuals know how to maximize their strengths and make them visible to others. You'll also identify some gaps— guaranteed. And that's all right. Either people don't see you as you want to be seen, or they see you in ways that aren't consistent with your desired image.

Here's how you can use this information:

> "The relationships that you nurture today will open tomorrow's opportunities. That's why it's important to surround yourself with people who are also hungry, passionate, smart, and good-hearted. You become your environment. What you draw near to is what you become."
>
> - Maureen Francisco

- Build missing brand attributes. This is an outstanding opportunity to build the brand attributes you lack but want to develop. These attributes are important to you—but for some reason, others don't see them as your primary brand attributes. Armed with that knowledge, you can take specific steps to address this gap.
- Avoid undesired brand attributes. Maybe you want others to see the jovial, approachable side of your personality—yet others have told you that you often seem reserved and serious. Assuming you have a reasonably accurate perception of yourself and you really *are* approachable and jovial despite what others may see (perhaps they don't get your sense of humor!), this is something you want to address head-on, as it's diametrically opposed to your goals.

> *"When you sign a contract with a label, you don't have much control over your own image, even in the music industry. You can't simply look like whatever you want when everyone else is promoting seduction and sexy. We don't need to change the entire industry. We just need options, authentic artists we can look up to."*
>
> *- Marika Siewert*

- Strengthen existing brand attributes. If you have a match, you have successfully aligned your desired image with the way others see you. Keep reinforcing the brand attributes you want at the core of your identity and that others identified with you.
- Consider new brand attributes. Others may have picked brand attributes for you that you didn't initially consider or expect, but that might appeal to you. It's not too late: decide if those attributes are desirable and consistent with your end goal and how you want to project yourself in the long run. It's always easier to enhance what's already working than to start from scratch.

How to Build a Personal Brand

Building a personal brand is within everyone's reach—you can start right now. Once you've carefully assessed and defined your brand, managing it is equally important: promoting, measuring and improving it. In other words, brands aren't built overnight. They take months, sometimes years to shape—though it might only take minutes to tarnish them! Brands are assets that must be attended to and cared for. There are four essential steps to constructing a personal brand, illustrated below in the "Brand Journey Wheel of Success":

- **KNOW:** defining your WHY
- **BUILD:** developing your brand plan

- **IMPLEMENT:** promoting and living your brand
- **REFINE:** measuring and improving your brand

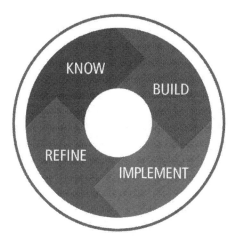

Figure 1 Brand Journey Wheel of Success

KNOW

What's your life purpose? This is the toughest question you'll ever have to answer. Having a clear sense of purpose is both empowering and liberating. Though it's core to our existence, few have successfully defined their purpose in life—what's often called "their WHY." Yet without it, we seem devoid of substance.

Everyone should have a sense of purpose that's personal; it's the critical distinction between living and existing. Rick Warren, pastor and author of *The Purpose-Driven Life,* says the antidote to spiritual emptiness is to "recognize what we have been given—creativity, talent, resources" and to use these gifts to make the world a better place. Many people lead successful lives by society's standards (they're rich or famous) but they're not fulfilled—emotionally, intellectually, or spiritually. How's that possible? How can they have so much and feel so empty? It's simple: they haven't found their true purpose in life.

> *"I want my work to be about the music, not image. I don't compromise what I do. It's about integrity and values. It's about being well aware of what you stand for."*
>
> *- Marika Siewert*

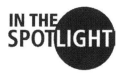
IN THE SPOTLIGHT

Got Five Minutes to Find out Your Life Purpose?

Adam Leipzig is the CEO of Entertainment Media Partners, former President of National Geographic Films and a former Senior VP of Walt Disney Studios. In his career, he has overseen more than 25 movies and produced more than 300 stage plays. Leipzig gave a simple yet memorable talk at TEDx Malibu entitled "How to Know Your Life Purpose in Five Minutes." At his 25th college reunion, he discovered that 80% of his classmates, typically financially well off and successful professionally, were unhappy with their lives. What were they missing? Leipzig told a captivated audience that answering these simple questions could help them find their life's purpose:

1. What do you love to do? What are you best at?
2. Who do you do it for? In other words, what audience do you serve? For example, a teacher would answer "children" and a public servant would answer "my community."
3. What do those people want or need? Why do they come to you?
4. How do they change or transform as a result of what you do for them?

The last three questions are outward facing, while the first is inward facing. When people ask you "what do you do?" at your next dinner event, tell them about the last three. And by the way, according to Leipzig, the most successful, fulfilled people tend to be those who focus most on the people they serve rather than on themselves. Finding our life purpose means understanding how we contribute to those around us. Who doesn't have five minutes to reflect on that?

People don't relate to *what* we do for a job or hobby; they relate to *why* we do it in the first place. They want to know what drives us—the story behind our interests and passions. The "why we do it" lies at the core of our existence and purpose. Without a clear understanding of our why, we're empty vessels, captains without maps. Here's what it takes to KNOW your personal brand statement:

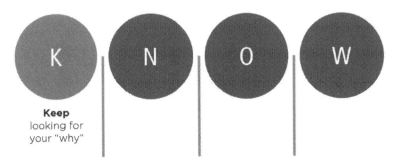

Keep
looking for
your "why"

1. **K**eep looking for your WHY. Never settle for a mediocre answer to this fundamental question: what I am here to accomplish? Keep looking deep inside for your answer until you find it—and it might take a lifetime to find. Some of us may want to use our professional success and personal influence to help others achieve their potential, inspiring them to push their limits. Some of us may want to dedicate ourselves to the pursuit of equality, justice or another admirable purpose. The quickest path to nowhere is a trip without meaning. You may not always have a map of how to get there, but you need an idea of where you're trying to go.

> *"I had the courage to leave the corporate world. I could have continued on this business path but I decided to take a risk and pursue something uncertain but more exciting, more fulfilling and establish myself in this new world of entertainment and creative art."*
>
> *- Melanie Kannokada*

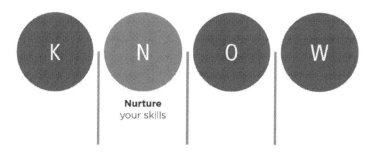

Nurture
your skills

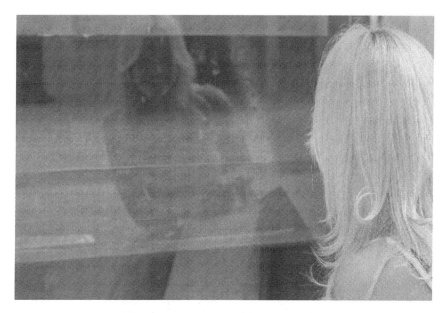

2. **N**urture your skills. What are your unique strengths and attributes? Learn your strengths so you can amplify them (and learn your weaknesses so you can overcome them). Find opportunities to build or enhance your skills. You might be good at connecting with others, at verbal or written communication, at convincing people or managing complex projects. No matter what your skills are, always look for ways to further develop and master them. These skills become an important part of your identity and how you project yourself.

In the case of Tina Fey, nurturing her writing, acting and comedy skills has been a big part of developing her brand identity; she's been rewarded by many Emmy Awards, Golden Globe Awards, Screen Actors Guild Awards and Writers Guild of America Awards. The talented comedian, known for her work on *Saturday Night Live, Mean Girls, Date Night* and the critically acclaimed *30 Rock,* studied at Second City, a well-known comedy training program. Her impersonations of Republican Vice Presidential nominee Sarah Palin became one of NBC's most-watched viral videos and contributed to Fey's fast-growing popularity. Known as "the thinking man's sex symbol" and for her legendary work ethic, Fey has focused diligently over the years on refining her skills to build a brand that's unique to her.

K N O W

Observe
your values
and beliefs

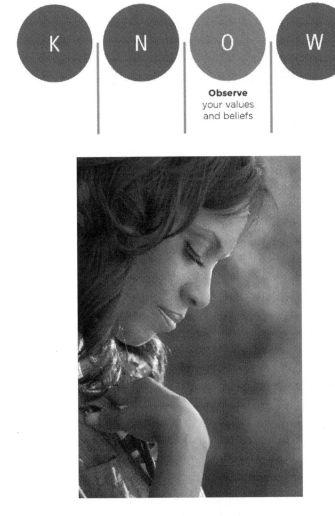

3. **O**bserve your values and beliefs. Make note of which ones best define you as an individual and as a community or family member. You may value mutual respect, open-mindedness to other ideas or ways of life, or transparency and trust in relationships. You may hold religious beliefs that shape your way of thinking and how you behave in everyday life. Be aware of these values—make them clear in the way you interact with others. Your values are an essential part of what you stand for, and how people see and interact with you. Values and beliefs are the most important part of projecting your personal brand.

> *"Always speak from the heart. Don't speak to impress. Be genuine and be authentic."*
>
> *- Brittany Dawn Brannon*

Television and film actress Jessica Alba might be number one on *Maxim's* "Hot 100 Babe List" and seen as a sex symbol by the general public, but her values and beliefs have shaped her reputation in an industry that can easily crush them. Her work in James Cameron's *Dark Angel,* the critically acclaimed *Sin City* and Marvel's blockbuster *Fantastic Four* propelled her toward a successful Hollywood career.

Alba's values were shaped early in life. She faced a range of physical maladies, including asthma, obsessive–compulsive disorder, partially collapsed lungs and pneumonia. Raised in a conservative Catholic Latin American family, she later developed liberal views. Alba is an ambassador for an organization that provides education to children in Africa; her charity work includes Clothes off Our Back, Habitat for Humanity, National Center for Missing and Exploited Children, and more. She's a vocal supporter of gay rights and protecting children from potentially dangerous chemicals in foods, toys and household products. As Alba has done, define your values and beliefs—and stay true to them.

> *"I am as much a family person as I am a professional woman. I maintain my family values in my career. You are not defined by your career but by who you are. Faith, grace and love are the foundation of our life. There is no point singing about love if you can't practice it at home."*
>
> *- Marika Siewert*

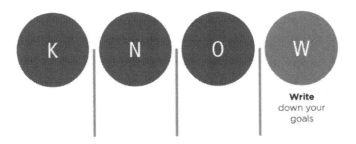

Write down your goals

4. **W**rite down your goals. Whether they're personal or professional, articulate them by committing them to a piece of paper. You may want to start your own company one day, explore your creativity, learn a new skill or lead a non-profit organization close to your heart. Once you've defined your short and long-term goals, you can enlist others' help in reaching them. You communicate them in your interactions with others. Your aspirations and ambitions say more about you as an individual than any other personal traits. Your goals become a central part of your brand.

"My biggest accomplishment has been to pursue my goals no matter what challenges were ahead. My story has inspired thousands. I received tons of emails, phone calls, and Facebook messages after the story of my participation in Miss Florida USA. I inspired so many other women with similar impairments or disabilities to be normal functioning adults with big dreams."

- *Connor Boss*

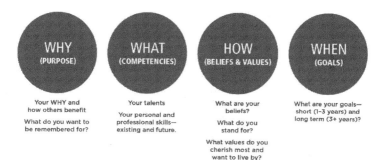

Writing a brand statement is a daunting task for most of us, but it's indispensable in building a personal brand. We can't accomplish much that matters in life without a clear sense of purpose. Knowing our "why" help us define who we are, what matters to us, what values and beliefs fuel us, what we hope to accomplish, and what we (as an individual and a brand) really stand for. Mark Twain said it best: "The two most important days in your life are the day you are born and the day you find out why." Know your "why" and watch it propel you forward.

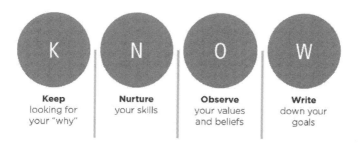

BUILD

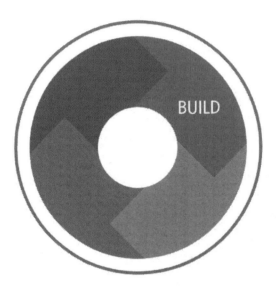

Now that you're on your way with a personal brand statement, let's define the brand strategies to help your brand gain recognition and traction. Failing to plan is planning to fail. We're not here to *wish* for an outcome . . . we're *driving* to that outcome.

The brand plan will help you BUILD your brand. What's in a brand plan? Here are the essentials:

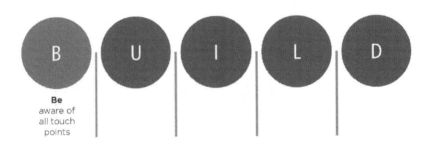

Be
aware of
all touch
points

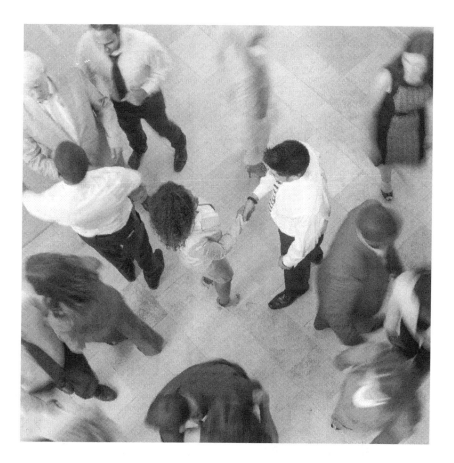

1. **Be** aware of all touch points. Touch points are the countless moments of contact with others that occur every day. Each touch point has the power to strengthen or weaken our brand: each form of interaction offers unique benefits and disadvantages to consider. Social media sites are known to provide fantastic reach, letting users expand their network or fan base in ways that far surpass any other communication vehicles—but too often they lack the personal touch of a real 1:1 human connection. Old-fashioned, face-to-face interactions at meetings or networking events give you the best opportunity to build your brand by establishing a personal connection with others, but this mode of communication doesn't scale well. In the end, there's

no right or wrong vehicle—just choices to make based on your brand objectives. Keep yourself informed of new channels of communication as they become available. Ask your friends and coworkers what they use most and why. Explore the vast number of touch points in your physical and online world-email, Facebook, networking events and so on-and determine which will work best to carry your message and support your personal brand.

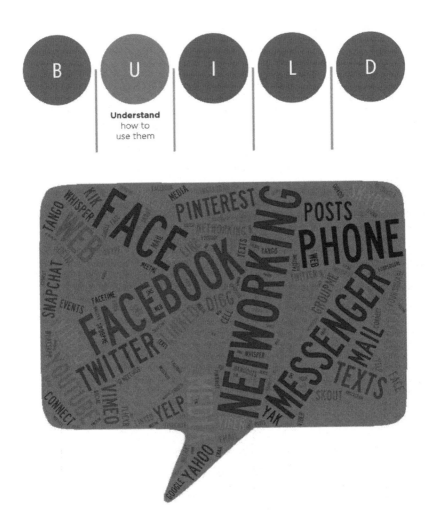

2. Understand how to use touch points. Figure out how to leverage them most effectively. Every touch point is different: managing your online presence and conducting yourself at public events require different skills and practical know-how. Thankfully, these skills can be learned and applied. Check for online resources, consult with people in your network who have mastered a particular skill. Create an elevator pitch so you can deliver key messages about yourself as a brand any time you get the chance.

> *"Image building is about highlighting what you like about yourself. I like to wear socially responsible clothing or give opportunities to young independent artists."*
>
> *- Marika Siewert*

Keira Knightley, the award-winning English actress known for her roles in *Pride and Prejudice* and *Pirates of the Caribbean,* knows how to use the full range of communication channels to support her personal branding efforts. And she knows how to leverage them to their fullest. In 2009 she appeared in a video called *Cut,* aimed at raising awareness of domestic abuse, for Women's Aid. To show her commitment to the cause, she travelled to Ethiopia on behalf of the Comic Relief charity. She posed for the American Library Association's "Read" campaign and became the face of both Chanel's perfume Coco Mademoiselle and an Amnesty International campaign to support human rights. She shares her every action, view and idea with fans on sites like www.keiraknightleyfan.com and kknightley.org/, on Facebook fan pages, on Twitter and on Instagram.

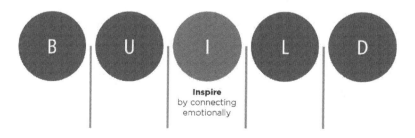

B U I L D

Inspire
by connecting
emotionally

3.   **I**nspire by connecting emotionally. People connect with others on an emotional level. To build a successful brand plan, connect with others—be relevant to them, touch their hearts, speak their language, and inspire them. And always consider how and where you communicate. It's much easier to really connect emotionally with someone face-to-face than by texting them.

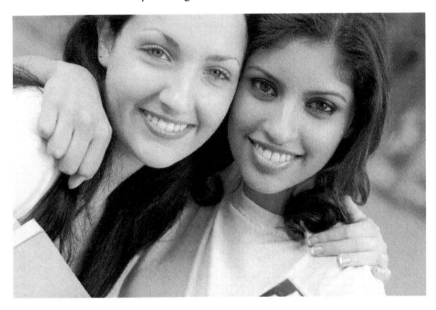

Comedian, host, actress, writer and producer Ellen DeGeneres has built a loyal audience of fans who fell in love with her highly entertaining, often quirky approach to television. Her gift at connecting emotionally with others has played a central role in her success on *The Ellen DeGeneres Show.*

Degeneres started her career by performing stand-up comedy at small clubs and coffee houses; she has now authored several books and opened her own record company, Eleveneleven. Her genuine personality and acute sense of humor led her to host the Academy Awards, Grammy Awards and the Primetime Emmys. On a more serious front, she was named by Secretary of State Hillary Clinton as Special Envoy for Global AIDS Awareness in late 2011. DeGeneres came out publicly as a lesbian in a 1997 appearance on *The Oprah Winfrey Show.* This sudden, bold announcement only reinforced her reputation for honesty and compassion: essential qualities for connecting emotionally with others.

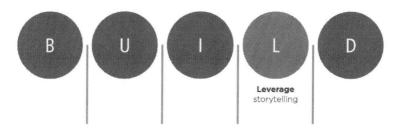

4. **L**everage storytelling. People love stories. They love to hear them. They'll love to hear yours too, if you tell it in a way that engages them, intrigues them, moves them.

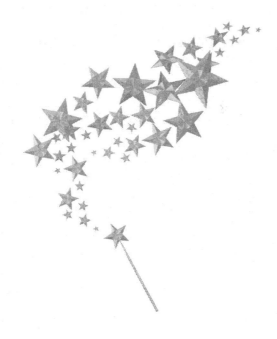

Everyone has a story: what's yours? Does it have a plot? A villain? What events shaped your life or took you on a different path than you'd planned? Ask yourself these questions and you'll be amazed at how presumably small events in your life—where you grew up, struggles family members or friends encountered, people who inspired you, events you witnessed—turn into amazing material for your story.

Here are the key ingredients of a good story: it should be simple, believable, compelling, unique and unexpected. Telling your story doesn't mean sitting down for a few hours. Successful people communicate who they are through story: they take just seconds to get someone's attention, connect with them emotionally, intrigue or inspire them, and leave people wanting to hear more and stay connected.

> *"Don't get involved with projects or people you don't want to be associated with. Protect your image. It's a valuable asset. More importantly, stay true to who you are. So think before you tweet. If it's not coming from a place of love, don't put it out there. You may regret it."*
>
> *- Susie Castillo*

As you build your personal brand plan, you especially want to develop your narrative in a way that's authentic. Oprah Winfrey's narrative is a big part of her brand, and it continues to inspire legions. This is a chance to tell your story in a way that connects with others and ensures the world sees you for who you really are. In a nutshell, build a brand worth promoting and people will find it worth loving. Guaranteed!

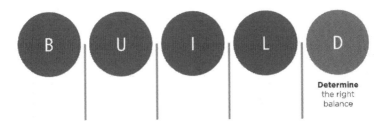

Determine the right balance

5. **D**etermine the right balance. An effective brand plan is carefully balanced so all aspects of your brand work together in a unified way. Some people prefer the intimacy of personal interactions. Others prefer (or need) to communicate their brand identity through online vehicles. Both are core elements of a strong brand plan; find the right balance and frequency based on your personal preferences and how aggressive your brand objectives are. How much is too much, or too little? For example, do you post or tweet hourly? Or simply daily? Do you blog semi-weekly or less frequently? Do you conduct in-person meetings weekly or more or less frequently? Do you attend networking events monthly? Every situation is unique, and finding the right balance is a personal choice. No matter what you do, it's essential to remain consistent at every interaction point and in your narrative so your image is identical at all times.

Apply the following recommendations by a top brand and marketing strategist to build a successful image that lasts and moves you forward.

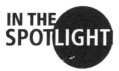
IN THE SPOTLIGHT

Top Five Recommendations by Brand and Marketing Strategist Karen Starns

With only slight adaptation, brand-building strategies of top organizations and corporations are applicable to cultivating your personal brand.

1. **Be intentional.** You have a brand whether you actively shape it or not. Understand your strengths and areas worthy of

---

development. Investing the time and energy to define your personal brand is empowering. Don't leave it to someone else!

2. **Uncover differentiation.** Brand relevance is helped by differentiation. Knowing what makes you different is necessary, but insufficient. Meaningful differentiation lives at the intersection of "different" and "matters to others." Find your differentiation and it will help you genuinely stand out.

3. **Embrace authenticity.** Be honest about who you are–whether strong, curious, expert, vulnerable, or all of the above. Eschew perfection. Demonstrate that you're trying to be the best version of you, not some idealized persona. Doing so will help drive the kind of connection that's key to brand building.

4. **Seek consistency.** Stay on message, keep reinforcing your story, and ensure people's experience of you ladders to the personal brand you want to build. When you start to get bored with your story is when it gains momentum. Stick with it—consistency will pay off!

5. **Consider associations.** Your relationships can energize your brand–or erode it. Be mindful of the individuals, organizations and groups you engage with. Ask yourself whether they're aligned with your values and beliefs. Focus on those that do, and those positive associations will help you establish your personal brand.

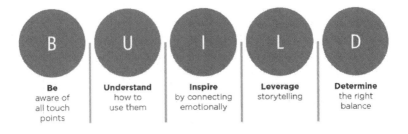

B	**U**	**I**	**L**	**D**
Be aware of all touch points	**Understand** how to use them	**Inspire** by connecting emotionally	**Leverage** storytelling	**Determine** the right balance

IMPLEMENT

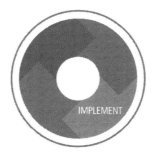

Once you've defined your plan, it's time to take action. Living and promoting your brand comes out of the preparation you've done up to this point. Coco Chanel understood better than anyone the power of bringing a brand to life and standing out in the process; as she put it, "In order to be irreplaceable, one must always be different." Every brand is different. Thankfully, there are best practices to follow when you IMPLEMENT your personal brand:

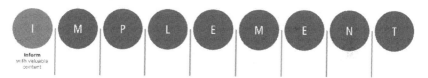

Inform
with valuable
content

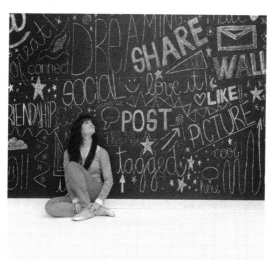

1. **I**nform with valuable content. Create content people want. In today's environment, content rules more than ever. There's value in content once it is sharable—either as text, visual, audio or video. You don't always need to create new content. You can simply contribute to conversations, ask questions, re-tweet articles, comment on posts, join a discussion, or share pictures, videos and stories that touched your heart.

What you post and *where* you post says a lot about you as a brand, so use good judgment. Know *when* to publish to get most impact: the secret to getting people's attention online is to post good content when they want it. Some great ideas never see the light of day because no one sees them. Engagement peaks tend to be consistent (Thursday, Friday, weekends) so focus on these times to post. See what works best for your audience, and adjust accordingly.

> *"Your Facebook account must always be clean. No risqué shoots or crazy partying. Be thoughtful about what you post. What I post on Facebook or what I write on my blog is the real me. I want others to see my inspirational, funny side. I never take myself too seriously. The best way to do that is to simply laugh about yourself and with others."*
>
> *- Connor Boss*

Be thoughtful about what you share with others. Find a balance between too little and too much: if you post too much, you can potentially get blocked, suspended or blacklisted. If you post too little, you can get lost in a sea of a billion interactions.

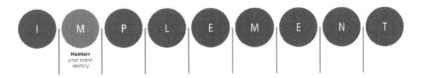

2. **M**aintain your brand identity. Don't weaken your brand by doing or saying things that get in the way of the brand you're building. We all remember Miley Cyrus's controversial, sexually charged performance at the 2013 MTV Video Music Awards that drew so much attention and press coverage.

> *"Every one of us is a brand ambassador. We all go to events and we can use these social opportunities to raise awareness about important issues to women and society."*
>
> *- Kristen Dalton*

When you meet new people, make eye contact, offer a firm handshake and a genuine smile, and exude a positive, inviting attitude. Don't present a particular image online if you're not conducting yourself that way in real life. Don't suggest that you're genuinely interested in others if you don't show that interest at business or social events. Stay true to your brand, even if it means getting less attention.

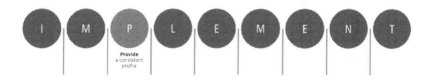

3. **P**rovide a consistent profile. Make sure your profile is complete, accurate and consistent across all online outlets you use. Make sure that your LinkedIn profile page matches your profile summary on Google+, Facebook or any other social network you use. Your profile should be optimized and indexed in Google, Yahoo and other top search engines so anyone can find it when they search for you. The more complete your profile, the easier it is for others to find you or get to know you. Tell who you are and what you care about—interests, hobbies, and passions—not just what you do or where you live. Attach a link to your profile or your website in your email signature. If you

make changes to your profile, make sure to update it everywhere else. Make sure it's always current: describe your most recent accomplishments, responsibilities, interests—and yes, even your relationship status. Be authentic at all times. People often give a distorted image of themselves in order to belong or impress. Stay true to who you are.

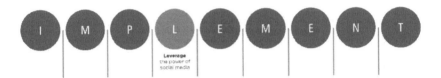

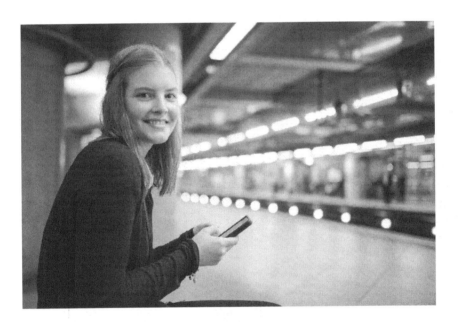

4. **L**everage the power of social media. Don't put all your eggs in the Facebook basket. Facebook is, and will likely remain, a very powerful connector (as is LinkedIn in your professional network), but don't ignore other popular personal and professional networking sites where you can build your online presence. YouTube, Pinterest, Instagram, Tumblr, Google+, Twitter and countless others being introduced every day also offer great network-building capabilities including

instant messaging, file sharing, photo/video editing, events/activity invites and more. See what others are using, and decide if those sites would be good for your networking too. Leverage your social media persona whenever possible.

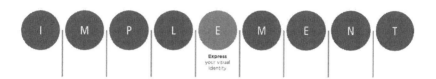

5. **E**xpress your visual identity. Consider scheduling a photo-shoot and hiring a reputable photographer to build a portfolio. No more half-cropped pictures of you from the last family reunion or selfies taken on a sunny day. Photographers are skilled in capturing your true personality and charisma. Use these pictures in your bio, on social networking sites, in your profile. Your profile is far more likely to be looked at if you have a picture.

Dress wisely for your photo shoot. Fashion, at its core, is a form of self-expression. Some may see it as superficial, but how we look and dress are important ways we express ourselves to the world around us. Yves Saint Laurent once said, "I have long believed that fashion's role was not only to make women beautiful but also to reassure them, give them confidence and allow them to assert themselves." When he retired, the celebrated designer added, "I understand that the most important encounter in life is the encounter with oneself."

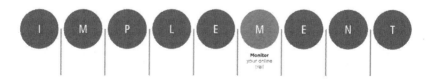

6. **M**onitor your online trail. Have you Googled yourself lately? If you haven't, consider doing so on a regular basis. See what comes up in major search engines like Google, Yahoo and Bing, and what people say

about you. Do you like what you see? Is it consistent with the image you want to project? Can your name be confused with someone else? Is the information about you accurate, consistent and current? Don't post questionable pictures or let others post them. If you post information online, think about keywords that might help others find you or associate with you. If you don't like what you find, consider hiring a reputation service like Reputation.com to clean up what's been posted about you.

> *"Don't put anything on social networks or the web that you don't want your grandkids to see. In today's digital age, everything you post or publish online will be around forever."*
>
> *- Brittany Dawn Brannon*

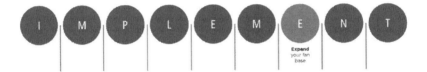

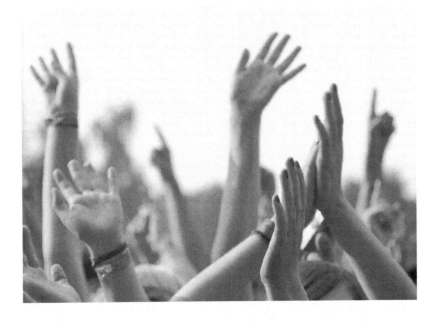

7. **E**xpand your fan base. Build a fan base through leading by example: if you inspire others by supporting a good cause or passion, encourage others to follow in your footsteps. Make yourself worth following. The larger your fan base, the greater your impact and influence. Don't fall in the trap of seeking a fan base for the sake of vanity. Think of it as an audience you're serving with valuable content and information.

Beyoncé, the American singer and actress known for her award-winning albums, has built a fantastic brand and an enormous fan base throughout her career. She has won many Grammy Awards over the years, regularly enjoying consecutive weeks at number one on the Billboard Hot 100 chart. She has sold over 100 million records worldwide as a solo artist and with Destiny's Child (her earlier group), making her one of the bestselling music artists of all time. With this track record, it's easy to see why she has such a vast fan base. Beyoncé's fan base is often called The Bey Hive, a purposeful misspelling of "beehive." (Its first name was "The Beyontourage," a blend of Beyoncé and entourage.)

Beyoncé is absolutely a brand, and a carefully managed one at that. Access her website at www.beyonce.com/ and you'll be invited to sign up for the newsletter and fan club to get her latest news sent directly to your inbox. She has over 13 million followers on Twitter who eagerly await her every word. She enjoys an equally large fan base on Facebook and Instagram. Although these figures are unusually large, Beyoncé's approach to building a fan base is standard, within everyone's reach.

> *"Omnipresence is everything. Be everywhere. Reach out to people and interact. Build a fan base. Facebook is an amazing way to do just that."*
>
> *- Heidi Forrest*

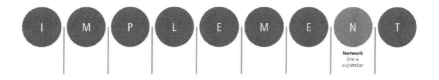

8. **N**etwork like a superstar. Networking is about opening new doors and building long-lasting relationships, not just short-term connections. It's also a necessity to reach almost any goal you set. Leverage your personal and professional connections wisely—your neighbors, friends, family members, sports buddies, college roommates, teachers, former colleagues and more. Tap into your network to land a new career opportunity, promote your business or conduct research. This is how business is done these days, and it's one of the most effective ways to find a job.

There are many ways to build a larger network. Most social networks are quite good at mining your inbox and identifying possible connections from your past or future based on your interests. They've figured out that the more connected you are, the more likely you are come back to their site. Build a support system you can tap into in pursuing your goals. Reach out to people who you want to be associated with, who you can learn from and who can impact your personal or professional life. Ask for introductions, referrals and advice. Return the favor and build goodwill along the way. It's never been easier to do. Choose quality over quantity any day, though—it's not a numbers game. The right contact can be more influential and supportive than thousands of unknown followers or "friends."

> *"I learned that you have to be proactive to really stand out. It gave me exposure to the not-for-profit world. It opened some doors. Everything else was my choice and my drive."*
>
> *- Melanie Kannokada*

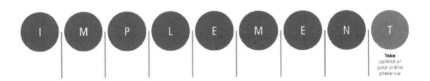

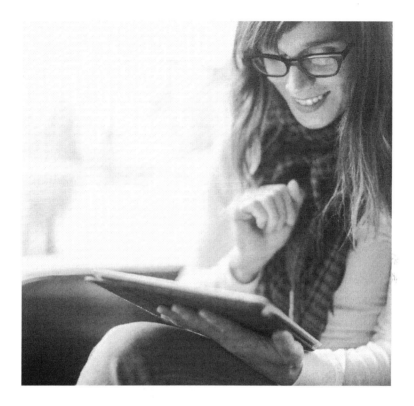

9. Take control of your online presence. Buy your domain name (www. yourname.com) from website registrars like GoDaddy.com for less than a movie ticket; build a personal website with your own content using WordPress or one of the many other web publishing tools. It's cheap and easy to do. If you need an extra hand, have someone build a site for you. Don't let others define your brand. Own your brand by owning the content others see: your profile, your visual identity, your content. Check out Michelle Sung Wie, the professional golfer whose prodigious golfing ability and charisma have made her one of the most influential athletes in women's sports. At the age of 10, she became the youngest-ever qualifier for a USGA amateur championship; she recently won her first major at the 2014 U.S. Women's Open. Wie, who turned professional shortly before her 16th birthday,

admits to being a serial Tweeter and Facebooker. She's sponsored by brand names including McDonald's, Nike, Kia Motors and Omega Watches. Wie also takes control of her online presence. She shares her life, favorite playlists, golf schedule, photos and videos on her website; she connects with fans and promotes her sponsors via Twitter, Facebook and email.

> *"I've met girls who changed themselves to become someone they are not to pursue their goals. Being authentic is knowing yourself well and sharing with others who you really are. Don't pretend to be someone you are not."*
>
> *- Connor Boss*

You don't need to be one of the most talented woman athletes to have your own website and social media channels. Apply the following recommendations by one of the top brand experts in the country and protect the brand you worked so hard to build.

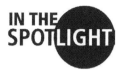

IN THE SPOTLIGHT

Top Five Recommendations by Brand Expert Michael Fertik

There's no question that we live in a brave new world of hyper-connectivity and instant awareness, all fueled by the rise of digital technologies. It's an incredible, exciting, if somewhat jarring, contrast to the not-so-distant past, in which your reputation was confined to the people who knew you. Your reputation was certainly known in your hometown, but didn't spread much beyond those borders (call it the predecessor of "What happens in Vegas, stays in Vegas").

Now, social media platforms like Facebook and Twitter mean we have an instant audience of friends and followers. Our LinkedIn profiles trumpet our professional accomplishments and signal our career aspirations and moves. Our search results reveal digital breadcrumbs and let anyone with a mobile phone to quickly form an opinion about who we are—even if it's based on outdated, incorrect or misleading results. In fact, about 70 percent of people don't look beyond the first four search results on page one of a Google search—and of those, about 32 percent only look at the first result. That's precisely why online reputation management is so critical. People are looking online and your reputation—good or bad—is cemented with a cursory glance. Here are five tips for branding yourself in a digital age:

1. **Audits are a good thing.** We shudder when we think of audits, no doubt traumatized by visions of the IRS and error-ridden tax returns. But in the context of your online reputation, an audit is an excellent idea. Search for your name using all the major search engines. Try variations that include your profession, your town and other identifiers people might use to find you (like "lisa smith

attorney"). Don't forget to check for images as well–visuals have a way of sticking with us. Take note of what you find. Are there any problematic results? What conclusions would people draw based on this information? What would you rather see reflected there? Set up free Google Alerts for fast updates when there's new content about you.

2. **Use social media more (and less).** Social media is a tool you should use strategically. That means first doing some cleanup on your personal accounts–remove posts that can be taken out of context, delete tweets that are borderline, untag yourself from photos that are unflattering. Lock down your privacy settings (but don't forget, you can never trust them to work completely, so share with care). Then open professionally oriented accounts that you'll use to show off your industry acumen. Even simply posting a relevant article with a question that invites dialogue– "What do you think?"–can be a useful way to demonstrate savvy.

3. **Look for the online mismatch.** Your online reputation is your digital personal brand. What are you trying to tell the world about yourself? One of the big mistakes I see is the online mismatch. You had an initial conversation with a recruiter where your enthusiasm for aerospace engineering resonated loud and clear. The recruiter checks you out online where a different passion–a love of snorkel-ling–dominates your results. Fatal? No–but it's a missed oppor-tunity to reinforce the messages you're sending offline. Imagine how much stronger an impression you would have made with results that reinforced your excitement about flight, space and engineering.

4. **Post considered content.** Luckily, it's relatively easy to start building a branded presence online. But you absolutely must use a considered approach as you go. Ask yourself before you create each piece of content how it will support your online image. Then start by creating your own website (www.YourName.com if it's available). Include educational and work accomplishments, a headshot designed to appeal to a business audience, links to your professional social media sites, etc. Create a blog that shows off your industry expertise–but only if you regularly update it.

5. **Borrow inspiration.** Keep an eye on those whose careers and professionalism you admire. Are they trying out new platforms with success? Changing up the tone of their blogs? What's working for them? There's no reason to be derivative, but there's also nothing wrong with a fresh infusion of inspiration from people you think are tops in the fields you care about.

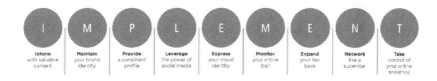

I	M	P	L	E	M	E	N	T
Inform with valuable content	**Maintain** your brand identity	**Provide** a consistent profile	**Leverage** the power of social media	**Express** your visual identity	**Monitor** your online trail	**Expand** your fan base	**Network** like a superstar	**Take** control of your online presence

REFINE

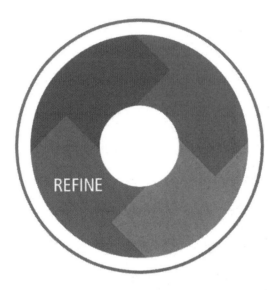

Be patient. Strong brands aren't built overnight. They're not static either. They evolve, grow and adapt. They can take months, even years to establish themselves. Rest assured: you can progress very quickly—in a matter of weeks—if you apply yourself. It doesn't always work the first time around. You learn, you try again . . . until it sticks. Don't give up—take one step at a time. Here's how to REFINE your brand:

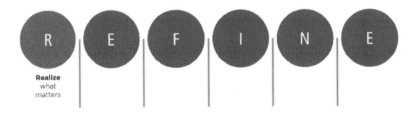

1. **R**ealize what matters. Determine what's important when deciding what to measure and improve. Not everything matters, and not everything matters equally. You may not care what strangers say about you on social media, but you might be quite interested in what your

professional network has to say. You may want to measure your social influence in terms of reach and perception.

> *"There is nothing better than human connections. In a world overwhelmed by technology and social media, I often encourage people to save money and go see their best friend across the country."*
>
> *- Marika Siewert*

At the end of day, though, there's only so much you can measure. As Einstein suggested, "Not everything that can be counted counts, and not everything that counts can be counted." Trust your instinct. Do you feel better about your image now? You may not be able to quantify it, but it matters greatly.

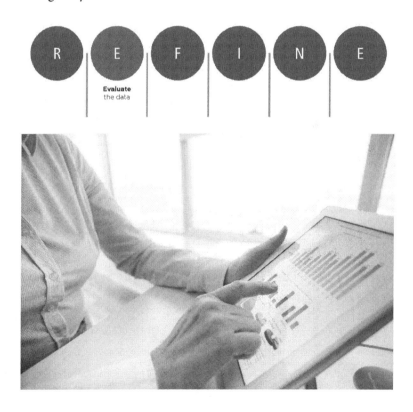

2. **E**valuate the data. There are many quick, effective ways to evaluate your brand data. Measure your reputation and influence using free or paid online services. These specialized services calculate likes, comments and reposts across your accounts like Facebook, LinkedIn and Twitter. Using their own proprietary methodology, they assess how your posts influence others. Check search engines to see how you rank. Choose keywords carefully in your profile so they show up over and over, boosting your visibility when someone conducts a keyword search.

You can also set up an alert system (Google Alerts is one) by entering search queries like your name and other keywords you want to monitor. You'll get email with the latest relevant Google results—web pages, newspaper articles or blogs—that match your search terms. Try to be as precise as possible; follow their tips to get the results you want. You can customize the frequency and volume of alerts, specific sources you want to track, and more.

Ask questions within your inner circle to learn what others see as your greatest strengths and weaknesses. Would they recommend you for a position at another company? Would they be willing to serve as a reference for you? Ask friends, colleagues and family members what they think about how your image has changed, and what they would do differently if they were in your shoes.

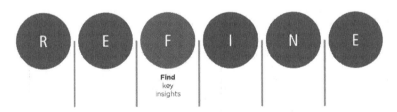

3. **F**ind key insights. Compile the data, organize it and look for possible trends (up, down or flat), potential gaps or inconsistencies between your goals and your current performance. Are you making progress in some areas but not others? Where are you lacking the most? Are

you getting closer to your end goal? If not, why not? What are the potential roadblocks? Look through your data carefully, reading between the lines to extract key insights.

> *"Don't be someone you're not. Your individuality makes you irreplaceable."*
>
> *- Heidi Forrest*

Look at the amazing Lila Tretikov, named to Forbes' list of "The World's 100 Most Powerful Women" in May 2014. Tretikov is Executive Director of the Wikimedia Foundation, a non-profit that provides access to knowledge through services like Wikipedia. This successful technology executive holds a number of patents in intelligent data-mapping and dynamic language applications. Russian-born, she moved to New York as a teenager and learned English while waitressing. She later studied Computer Science and Art at the University of California, Berkeley, where she conducted research work in machine learning. With such a remarkable background, it's safe to assume that when Tretikov looks at data, she's able to generate key insights.

> *"Prioritize. You can do anything you want in life but you don't do it all at once."*
>
> *- Melanie Kannokada*

Rest assured: you don't need a Computer Science degree or a list of patents to figure out where you land in Google search results or whether you're increasing your influence with a wider number of fans in your social networks. Next time you feel challenged, ask yourself: what would Tretikov do?

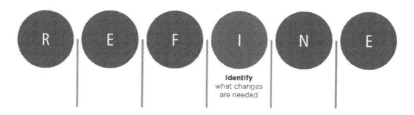

R E F I N E

Identify
what changes
are needed

4. **I**dentify what changes are needed. Decide if you need to adjust your brand plan based on the key insights you generated. Determine what's working, what's not, and why. Do you need to adjust the ways you promote and live your brand? Should you invest time in building a stronger online presence? Do you need a larger fan base to carry your message? Do you need to improve your image with a particular audience? Pick one or two focus areas; stick to those until your efforts pay off.

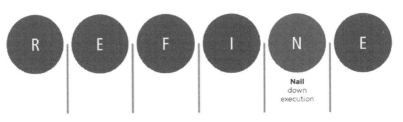

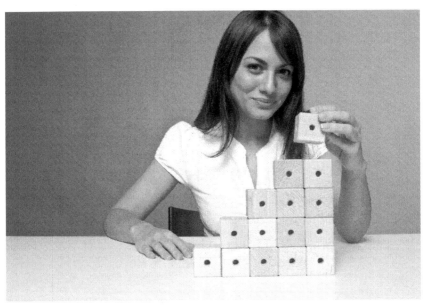

5. **N**ail down execution. Execution is everything. You may have the best plan, but if you' re not following through and making needed changes to your brand, you won't realize the benefits in your personal or professional environments. Work to remedy anything you think

might negatively impact your reputation. Once you've identified what changes you need to make, implement these improvements until you get the results you're after. Execute flawlessly.

J. K. Rowling is best known as the dazzling British author of *Harry Potter,* the best-selling book series in history (with over 400 million copies sold) and the basis for the highest-grossing film series in history. She conceived the idea for the Harry Potter series on a train delayed between Manchester and London. It took several years—during which her mother passed away and Rowling herself got divorced and struggled as a jobless single mother living on government benefits—until the first novel was finished. Today she's an international literary icon and an inspiration to generations of Harry Potter fans.

Rowling is also a wizard at managing her brand identity and reputation. She has taken legal action against the unauthorized use of photographs and grotesque rumors about her life. Her appearances and online presence, including her official website, are carefully orchestrated and flawlessly executed to support her unique, captivating personal brand.

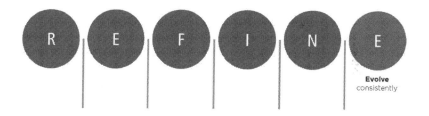

6. **E**volve consistently. You've made some changes and improved your personal brand. Are you done? Not quite. To sustain these benefits, you must consistently evaluate how you do and correct your course as needed. Your brand must evolve with you as your needs and goals change. It's a journey that never really ends—refining your brand so it's always aligned with your priorities.

> *"Life taught me to be mentally strong, build a strong protective shell and pay attention to who you are and want to be. It takes a lifetime to build a reputation and one second to ruin it."*
>
> *- Brittany Dawn Brannon*

Brand building is a lifelong journey. In some ways, you just took your first steps by reading this chapter. Treat personal branding like any other area in your life: seek to understand what works for you and what doesn't. In the end, we can't improve what we can't measure. Measurement is key to continuous improvement. The only way to improve and strengthen your personal brand is to determine what really matters, capture and analyze data, generate insights to understand what changes you need to make, and implement new action plans.

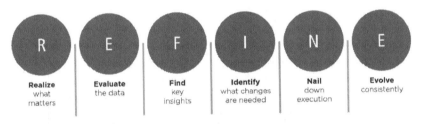

R	E	F	I	N	E
Realize what matters	**Evaluate** the data	**Find** key insights	**Identify** what changes are needed	**Nail** down execution	**Evolve** consistently

Follow the personal branding principles in this chapter (summarized below) and you'll have what you need to build a powerful, authentic image that propels you forward.

Know
- [ ] Keep looking for your "why"
- [ ] Nurture your skills
- [ ] Observe your values and beliefs
- [ ] Write down your goals

Build
- [ ] Be aware of all touch points
- [ ] Understand how to use them
- [ ] Inspire by connecting emotionally
- [ ] Leverage storytelling
- [ ] Determine the right balance

Implement
- [ ] Inform with valuable content
- [ ] Maintain your brand identity
- [ ] Provide a consistent profile
- [ ] Leverage the power of social media
- [ ] Express your visual identity
- [ ] Monitor your online trail
- [ ] Expand your fan base
- [ ] Network like a superstar
- [ ] Take control of your online presence

Refine
- [ ] Realize what matters
- [ ] Evaluate the data
- [ ] Find key insights
- [ ] Identify what changes are needed
- [ ] Nail down execution
- [ ] Evolve consistently

Although these four practices (Know-Build-Implement-Refine) are vital to establishing a strong, lasting personal brand image, we all value those practices differently because of our individual skills or gaps. I discovered that most women value knowing their purpose in life (Know) in order to build a strong image. This is true across the board, no matter their background or demographic segment. They also value measuring and improving how others see them (Refine), followed by having a clear plan to build their image (Build) and promoting themselves (Implement), all practices more valued by younger generations.

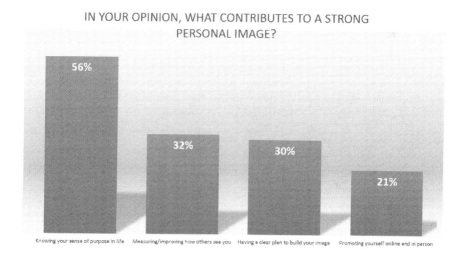

IN YOUR OPINION, WHAT CONTRIBUTES TO A STRONG PERSONAL IMAGE?

56% — Knowing your sense of purpose in life
32% — Measuring/improving how others see you
30% — Having a clear plan to build your image
21% — Promoting yourself online and in person

In the world of brands, perception is often reality. Your personal brand lets you shape others' perceptions of who you are, your life purpose, your story and the values you stand for. Just as brands reinvent themselves and mature over time, your brand should reflect where you are in your life, personally and professionally. We change our aspirations, gain new experiences, accept new life challenges, and evolve in our thinking. Oprah Winfrey's brand has gone through many iterations over the years; it's far more polished now than in her early years. Follow these four main steps—KNOW, BUILD, IMPLEMENT and REFINE—and watch your personal brand take off. You're well underway to a strong, authentic brand that will influence and inspire others.

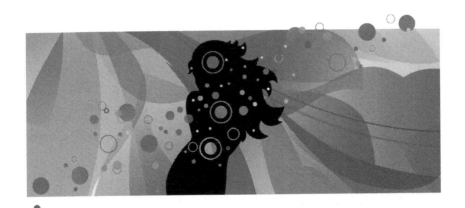

*"Do you love me
because I'm beautiful,
or am I beautiful
because you love me?*

**- Oscar Hammerstein II,
American Theatrical Producer**

CONCLUSION

In her inspiring song *"Beautiful,"* artist Christina Aguilera invites women to look inside to find their inner beauty, ignoring the judgment of others: *"I am beautiful no matter what they say, words can't bring me down, I am beautiful in every single way."* My daughter Anaïs mentioned this song to me as a sort of national anthem for young women. Anaïs and Aguilera are right: you are beautiful, no matter what. In earlier chapters, we established that beauty isn't found in stereotypes where only thin, tall or fit is glorified.

Too many women still suffer from low self-esteem, comparing their looks to superficial physical standards. In doing this, they miss opportunities to celebrate their true splendor. Fearing rejection and wanting to blend in, many have focused on the outer shell as a sign of self-worth. They let others define them.

> *"People sense real beauty. It's an energy you can feel. You can sense if you are captivated by that person. Most people don't have a clear sense of what beauty is and seek external validation."*
>
> *- Melanie Kannokada*

From childhood to adulthood, society has conditioned us to think that how we look is more than important than who we are. This grossly limited—not to mention unattainable—definition of beauty has plagued generations of women for too long. It's time for it to end. We have only limited control over our physical features or our personal circumstances, like the environment we grew up in, the people who shaped our early years. But we CAN control how we use and care for our body. We can also control of how we develop our mind, how we strengthen our heart and how we shape our image. More importantly, we have full control over how we perceive ourselves and how we become the best version of ourselves.

Embracing Our Human Instincts

Some argue that the concept of physical beauty should be downplayed or disregarded altogether. But dismissing physical appearance as inconsequential would be naïve and ill-advised. When asked, "What makes a woman beautiful?," "personality" and "a nice figure/body" are equally important to most women. Although women and men agree that personality is by far what makes a woman most beautiful, not so surprisingly perhaps, men also see beauty in the way women express it physically. We can't deny human nature. As humans, sight remains our most keen and decisive sense. It's how we—regardless of gender—process information, make decisions and explore the world around us.

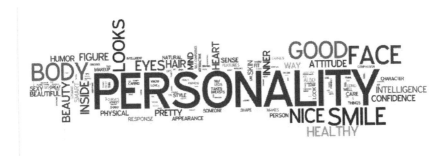

Figure 1. Word Cloud "What makes a woman beautiful?" (Men only)

Many species rely on visual markers of genetic fitness as signs that potential offspring will be healthy—so to some extent appearance does matter, consciously or not. Aesthetics will always be relevant in attracting a mate. It's a natural survival instinct.

In one of my favorite books, *The Upside of Irrationality: The Unexpected Benefits of Defying Logic*, Duke University Professor Dan Ariely explains that in society, beauty tends to define our place in the social hierarchy along with our mating potential. In Ariely's study of speed-dating participants, less attractive people put more emphasis on nonphysical attributes, while attractive people emphasized the physical.

Ariely's findings made me wonder—as I am sure you do too—what drove participants to act in these ways. Ariely, who experienced an accident when he was young that left him badly scarred, argues that we scorn what we can't have as being not-that-good in the first place, moving the scale of perfection closer to our own imperfect selves. People just change the priority of attributes they care about.

As humans and social creatures, we have a basic need to be accepted that's driven by evolutionary biology and culture. So it's only natural that women who admire beauty of all kinds would want to find beauty in themselves as well. We're conditioned to believe that what pleases the eye is more enjoyable and yields greater pleasure.

> *"Being beautiful inside and out starts with the heart shining through. You are beautiful inside when you use beauty for good and invest in others."*
>
> *- Brittany Dawn Brannon*

Many women have an inherent desire to feel they're attractive and beautiful. I'm not suggesting that caring for your appearance is wrong. This book has offered worthy suggestions to look and feel your best. There's overwhelming evidence that physical appearance can be a powerful asset. People who are perceived—or who perceive themselves—as "attractive" tend to be more successful and end up with more power and status in today's society. The more valued we are by our own communities, the better our self-image, and vice versa. How we feel about our appearance affects our self-esteem, confidence level and by extension our ability. It affects what we believe ourselves capable of. If channeled wisely, it can be a healthy source of empowerment and personal strength.

You Are Beautiful, No Matter What

One of the world's most beautiful temples lies in the southern portion of the Indochina Peninsula in Southeast Asia, in Cambodia. The Hindu temple, built in the 10th century, is named after the ancient capital: *Banteay Srei,* meaning "Citadel of Beauty" or "Citadel of Women." The reliefs are so delicate, so fine and small, that it's assumed they could only have been created by a woman's hand. Many words on the inscriptions are impossible to decipher, even to Buddhist monks who attempt to interpret inscriptions carved over a thousand years ago. I often wonder what these words would tell us if they were written by women. They might speak of ancient Hindu legends. They might also invite us to go far beyond the physical splendor of the temple and see the spiritual beauty that lies within it. In some ways, *Banteay Srei* reminds me that being beautiful is about knowing who you really are, regardless of what you see, hear and are made to believe. Nature's wonders—whether *Banteay Srei* or people themselves—are so much more than their outward appearance suggests. Let's reject the false belief that a woman's worth is just tied to her looks—without becoming indifferent about how we look. Everything in life calls for moderation and a careful balance. Daughter of Aerosmith's Steven Tyler and model Bebe Buell, actress Liv Tyler once said: "There is no definition of beauty, but when you can see someone's spirit coming through, something unexplainable, that's beautiful to me." Tyler's view is shared by many. When a woman is known and valued based on her looks, it only diminishes her own self-perception. Learn to love WHO YOU ARE without relying on your physical appearance, but without disregarding its place in the human condition. This graphic shows that the more you rely on yourself (rather than others) to define your own beauty, the more fulfilled you're likely to be.

> *"True beauty comes from loving yourself. You can't love others if you don't love yourself. If you love the person you are, love others and live by the golden rule of treating others as you would like to be treated, then you are truly beautiful."*
>
> - *Susie Castillo*

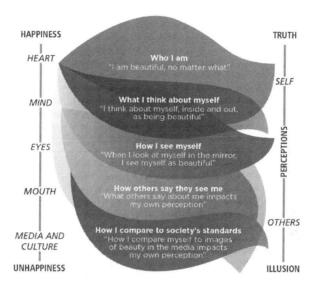

If our mind tricks us into a distorted perception of self—whether physical, emotional, intellectual or spiritual—or if we rely on others in seeing ourselves, we set ourselves up for heartache and unhappiness. Many women judge themselves harshly and inaccurately. When they look in a mirror (literal or figurative) they often pick apart their flaws instead of focusing on things they love about themselves. The reality is that women are far more beautiful than they think.

Dr. Elizabeth Lindsey is the first Polynesian Explorer and female Fellow in the history of the National Geographic Society. She's also an internationally recognized expert in the emergent field of cultural intelligence. She tells powerful stories about the various meanings of beauty across different cultures:

I lived among women who have never seen a mirror. No mirrors. They perceive themselves as beautiful, luscious, and sensuous. In fact, they have no doubt about it. And I'm referring to 90-year olds who flirted wildly with my crew, toothless women with breasts to their waists. They remind me that beauty is a state of mind. . . .

In other cultures elders are revered because they are wealthy—rich with life experience and wisdom. In western society we abhor the notion of aging, we shove it away, refuse to go near it, do everything we can to remain as youthful as possible. We equate beauty with youth, an illusory and disempowering myth. I believe in optimizing life—choosing a healthy lifestyle, teeming with vibrant choices, which includes feeling and looking your best. I love beauty. Beauty, grace, elegance—all are qualities much needed in our current society. But I maintain a much broader definition of beauty than the superficial focus that we tend to maintain.

To Lindsey, a beautiful woman is "a woman who is true to herself, who is wise, self-loving, which includes self-accepting, self-nurturing."

> *"The most common misconception today is to confuse beauty with pleasing physical features and sex appeal. Being beautiful inside and out means so much more than this simplistic view. It is the willingness to be open to the world and a choice all women must make to shine through and from within."*
>
> *- Connor Boss*

A new way of looking at beauty is emerging thanks to healthy, strong, confident women who are tremendously successful in their personal and professional lives. In Colbie Caillat's video "Try," the Grammy Award-winning singer-songwriter calls attention to unfair beauty ideals. The video begins with Caillat and a range of actors in full makeup; it ends with them all makeup-free, without the help of hair stylists or makeup artists.

"Try" isn't really about the excessive use of Photoshop or makeup. Rather, it's about losing yourself in the face of arbitrary standards about beauty and worth. Each woman is beautiful in her OWN WAY: in her natural state or not. Some women enjoy wearing makeup, styling their hair and dressing up— others don't.

When asked to think about the time, money and energy they expend on beauty and their overall motivations for doing so, the majority of women say they do it for themselves or to boost their confidence.

Most men believe that women's motivations are slightly different, more about external validation than for themselves. Although they agree that one of the primary reasons women care about being beautiful is boosting their confidence, men see the primary reason as to "stay looking young" and to attract a potential partner.

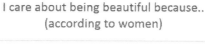

I care about being beautiful because..
(according to women)

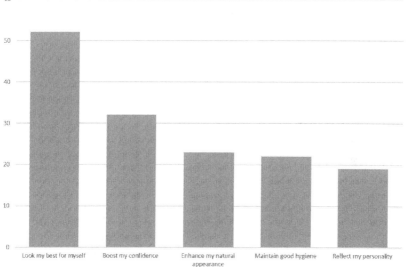

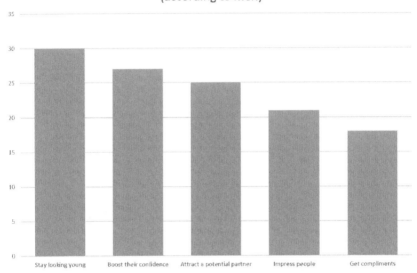

Women care about being beautiful because they want to...
(according to men)

There's nothing wrong with wanting to look your best for yourself, to boost your confidence, for a date with someone special or an important meeting at work. It's *WHY* you do it that matters. If you make a choice for yourself or someone you love, you're on the right track. If you decide based on a need to meet arbitrary standards or under pressure, you're setting yourself up for disappointment. You also want to explore other non-physical ways to express your beauty.

The campaign "You Are Beautiful," started by Matthew Hoffman (you-are-beautiful.com), inspires women "to create moments of positive self-realization," celebrating the idea that "each individual is intriguing, complex and beautiful." I couldn't have said it any better.

How often have we met attractive people, only to learn over time that their beauty fades because of their actions towards us or others? Likewise, we often meet people who don't at first appear particularly attractive, but whose kindness, attitude and actions make them suddenly beautiful in our eyes. How we treat others, how we interact with our community, the strength of our character, are hallmarks of true nature and true *beauty*. To redefine beauty, learn to emphasize intellectual achievement, personality traits, moral strength, strong values and other human qualities that set you apart.

> *"Being beautiful inside and out means that you don't just have a pretty face and expect things in return for standing in front of a camera. It means spreading your inner beauty outward and inspiring everyone who you meet by making a difference in your community and truly caring for other people."*
>
> *- Heidi Forrest*

Remind yourself: "I am a good child, parent or sibling," "I am a kind neighbor," "I am a dedicated and compassionate spouse," "I am a faithful friend," and so on. Change your outlook—in doing so, you can change yourself!

Cultivating Imperfection

Let's usher in a concept of beauty far deeper than our eyes can see. One that doesn't bend to social pressure and doesn't fade with time. Let's embrace the natural physical diversity embodied by women and men around the world. Let's encourage people to be comfortable in their own skins, minds and hearts . . . celebrating individuality and avoiding the traps of conformity. What we may see as a flaw or imperfection, others may see as perfect or unique. Often the things we don't like about ourselves are the very things others treasure . . . and what make us beautiful. "Everything has beauty," said Confucius, "but not everyone sees it."

> *"Being beautiful inside and out is loving who you are and loving others. When you know how beautiful you are, you start shining. It's more about how you carry yourself than what make up you are wearing. We become beautiful outside when we are beautiful inside."*
>
> *- Marika Siewert*

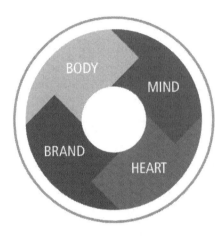

Being "*magnifique* inside & out" is a mindset. It's a statement—a pledge to challenge the status quo. It's a more fulfilling approach to life. Of course, it's easier said than done. Disenchantments are inevitable, the roadblocks are many—but the path forward is clear. It lies in the careful synergy of physical, mental, emotional, brand-building qualities covered in this book—qualities whose sum is much greater than its parts.

Though we may have a lot in common, we're all different, and in that we find comfort. Perfection never existed and never will. If it did, how boring our world would be! Character building has always been about cultivating imperfection. It's as essential as oxygen is to life. We must appreciate who we are regardless of what others think. We must celebrate what makes us unique and different. In the end, the *real* you is how you define yourself. We all know intuitively that real happiness comes from within. The ability to be yourself: this is what brings happiness and peace to the heart and soul.

> "*Success to me is how many lives I have impacted and made better.*"
>
> - Maureen Francisco

Keys to Unlock the Power of Beauty

In this book, we identified the key ingredients of inner and outer beauty—a healthy body, a powerful mind, an authentic image, and a strong heart—and how to develop these ingredients:

I invite you to step into the light with courage and confidence, using this book as your personal guide. Something remarkable will happen: your mind and heart will shine for the world to discover how beautiful you are—inside and out. The key to realizing dreams and unlocking the power of beauty isn't hidden in any magical formula or breakthrough discovery. It's already in each of us. When you find out or simply rediscover how truly beautiful you are, share your story with others.

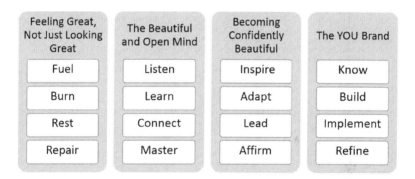

Feeling Great, Not Just Looking Great	The Beautiful and Open Mind	Becoming Confidently Beautiful	The YOU Brand
Fuel	Listen	Inspire	Know
Burn	Learn	Adapt	Build
Rest	Connect	Lead	Implement
Repair	Master	Affirm	Refine

In the end, I firmly believe that being beautiful is—and has always been—about love: love of oneself and love of others. A woman who knows she's loved and valued is a woman blossoming. To answer Oscar Hammerstein II's question, "Do you love me because I'm beautiful, or am I beautiful because you love me?" the answer is definitely the latter.

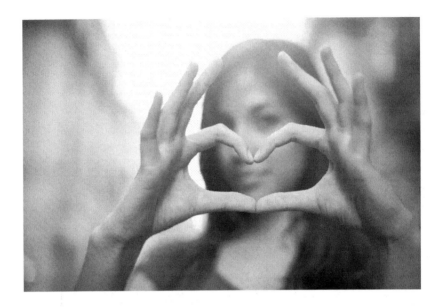

Love is what connects us all as human beings. We are "*magnifique inside & out*" when we love and are loved in return. French poet and aviator Antoine de Saint-Exupéry had it right in a touching book that's been translated into more than 250 languages. As he wrote in *Le Petit Prince (The Little Prince)*, "*Voici mon secret. Il est très simple: on ne voit bien qu'avec le cœur. L'essentiel est invisible pour les yeux.*" Translation: "It is only with the heart that one can see rightly. What is essential is invisible to the eye."

BIOS OF KEY CONTRIBUTORS

(IN ORDER OF APPEARANCE)

Susan M. Kleiner

Dr. Susan M. Kleiner is a titan in sports nutrition. A renowned authority on eating for strength, endurance, power and speed, her bestselling POWER EATING® program has reshaped the lives of thousands. Dr. Kleiner is the co-founder and co-CEO of the newly launched venture, Vynna®, LLC, an evidence-based, female-centric sports nutrition brand owned and operated completely by women, and a subsidiary of Vitargo Global Sciences, LLC. Dr. Kleiner has been consultant to many professional sports teams, including the Seattle SuperSonics, Storm, and Seahawks, Cleveland Browns and Cavaliers and Miami Heat. She has worked individually with NFL, MLB and NBA All Stars, NBA Championship Finals MVPs, and NBA Rookie of the Year, as well as Olympian medalists and world champions. Dr. Kleiner is the author of seven books including the international bestseller *POWER EATING®* (Human Kinetics, 2014), now in its fourth edition, as well as *The Oxygen Diet Solution* (Robert Kennedy Publisher, 2012), *The Good Mood Diet* (Springboard Press, 2007), and *The POWERFOOD Nutrition Plan* (Rodale Press, 2005). She has also authored *The POWER EATING® AND FITNESS LOG* (Get Pumped, 1999), *Be Healthier Feel Stronger Vegetarian Cookbook* (Macmillan, 1997),

High-Performance Nutrition: The Total Eating Plan to Maximize Your Workout (Wiley, 1996), and *The High-Performance Cookbook* (Macmillan, 1995). A scientist and author of professional research journal articles, she is one of the foremost nutrition authorities on eating for strength, a national columnist and speaker on the subject of nutrition, sports and fitness. Dr. Kleiner's credentials include a PhD in Nutrition and RD, FACN, CNS, FISSN certifications and honors.

Linda Melone

Linda Melone, CSCS, is a well-published health and fitness writer, certified personal trainer and a National Strength and Conditioning Association (NSCA) Certified Strength and Conditioning Specialist. Her background includes a degree in foods and nutrition. Her articles regularly appear in print publications ranging from *AARP The Magazine* to *Family Circle, Prevention, Oxygen, Better Homes & Gardens,* as well as online at Health, Shape, Livestrong, Today, iVillage, NextAvenue, Prevention, MensFitness and many others. In addition to her freelance work, Melone also writes a weekly blog and newsletter focused on the fitness and weight-loss concerns of women over 50. She is the author of the new eBook, *Break Up With Your Fat After 50: A Step-by-Step Guide to An Ageless Body,* available on her website, www.LindaMelone.com.

Bobby Bakshi

Bobby is the Chief Inspiration Officer of Resonant Insights LLC—a strategic consulting firm focused on evoking the best in brands and the people who bring them to life. Bakshi is a public speaker and an advocate of conscious culture creating brand value. He speaks and trains on the subject of purpose driving individual and organizational success. His book *The 101% You: Seven Steps to Creating the Life of Your Choice* is based on the metaphor of how he tackled a leadership ropes course exercise. Bakshi believes we all have had peak events that we can leverage to overcome our current challenges and turn them into opportunities for growth. Before launching his own practice, he held management positions at global corporations including eight years at Microsoft where he was responsible for a deeper understanding of customers. He designed and led an international people development program for the central marketing group at Microsoft that set the course for a strategic internal initiative. A global citizen, Bakshi lived and worked in many parts of the world. He has an MBA from Loyola University Chicago and is skilled in several organizational development practices. He lives in the Seattle area with his wife, two daughters and son. He strives to fully live his mission: to inspire people to be their best with compassion, courage and abundance.

Robyn Hatcher

Robyn Hatcher is an author and communication skills expert who brings more than 17 years of experience to her position as Founder and Principal of SpeakEtc., a boutique communication and presentation-skills training company. Hatcher recently launched her first book, *Standing Ovation Presentations* (Motivational Press, 2013), a complete presentation skills guide that contains a unique communication-style system called ActorTypes. Over the course of her career, she has helped thousands of business professionals improve their presentations and conduct successful interviews and interpersonal communication. Her clients have included C-suite executives and entrepreneurs as well as academics and human services professionals. Her corporate client roster has included Fortune 500 companies and noteworthy brands, including Lifetime Television, Jones New York, AXA, Jet Blue, Deloitte & Touche and Merrill Lynch. Prior to founding her own consultancy, Hatcher worked as a professional actress, appearing on stage in New York and surrounding regions, as well as in television commercials and dramas.

Christine Serb

Christine is passionate about helping women pursue their dreams and has dedicated her career to bringing savvy and goal-oriented women together to influence the world through the exploration of both inner and outer beauty. Serb is the head of casting for Pageants NW LLC., which produces the Miss Washington USA, Miss Washington Teen USA, Miss Idaho USA, Miss Idaho Teen USA, Miss Montana USA and Miss Montana Teen USA. Miss USA is part of the Miss Universe Organization, a partnership of NBC Universal and Donald Trump. In this capacity, she has successfully recruited and coached hundreds of talented and ambitious young women looking to pursue their careers, personal and humanitarian goals and seeking to improve the lives of others. Originally from Orange County, California, and of Romanian heritage, Serb values the importance of family, tradition and positive relationships. Her approach to life is both realistic and highly optimistic. Her coaching approach is based on a core set of proven confidence-building principles that have helped countless women unleash their full potential and prepare them for life challenges, both in personal or professional surroundings. Serb is also the Founder and Principal of Beautiful Inside Out LLC, a Seattle-based firm dedicated to building the new generation of women leaders through personal development and leadership workshops and personalized life coaching and mentoring.

Karen Starns

For more than 20 years, Starns has been an industry leader in technology marketing with depth in branding, advertising and media, demand generation, CRM, digital marketing, strategic partnerships, channel programs, loyalty programs, and product launches. She is most known for brand strategy, consumer marketing, and developing high performing teams. Starns joined Amazon in 2014 to build a new global advertising function responsible for advertising and media planning. Her work cuts across the entire Amazon portfolio–from Amazon to Kindle, Prime to Fire tablets, and Fire TV to Fire phone. She has directed brand efforts across three key pillars: definition, design and delivery. Having led the Global Brand Strategy practice for Microsoft, Starns developed the portfolio strategy for emerging and established brands–Microsoft, Bing, MSN, Microsoft Dynamics, Office, Exchange, SharePoint, Windows,

Windows Phone and Microsoft CRM. While leading consumer marketing for Bing and MSN, she was credited with developing and driving the
"Bing it On" Google compete campaign, the most effective marketing
campaign in the history of Bing which achieved more than 25 million
visits to bingiton.com and drove measurable impact on perception and
search share. She has also been an advisor to start ups and SMBs, helping them hone their brand and marketing strategies. Prior to 12 years
at Microsoft, she held leadership positions at Great Plains Software and
Compaq Computer after getting her start in small technology firms.
A top technology leader and speaker on brand and advertising, Starns
is currently co-authoring her first book on disciplined leadership. She
earned a Bachelor's of Business Administration in marketing from The
University of Texas at Austin.

Michael Fertik

Michael Fertik founded Reputation.com with the belief that people and
businesses have the right to control and protect their online reputation
and privacy. A futurist, Michael is credited with pioneering the field of
online reputation management (ORM) and lauded as the world's leading cyber-thinker in digital privacy and reputation. Fertik was most
recently named Entrepreneur of the Year by TechAmerica, an annual
award given by the technology industry trade group to an individual
who embodies the entrepreneurial spirit that made the U.S. technology
sector a global leader. He is a member of the World Economic Forum
Agenda Council on the Future of the Internet, a recipient of the World
Economic Forum Technology Pioneer 2011 Award; through his leadership, the Forum named Reputation.com a Global Growth Company in
2012. Fertik is an industry commentator with guest columns in *Harvard
Business Review, Reuters,* Inc.com and *Newsweek.* Named a LinkedIn
Influencer, he regularly blogs on current events as well as developments
in entrepreneurship and technology. Fertik frequently appears on na-
tional and international television and radio, including the BBC, *Good
Morning America, Today Show, Dr. Phil, CBS Early Show,* CNN, Fox,

Bloomberg, and MSNBC. He is co-author of the bestselling book, *Wild West 2.0,* and author of the upcoming book, *The Reputation Economy,* to be published by Crown Business in March 2015. Fertik founded his first internet company while at Harvard. He received his JD from Harvard Law School.

KEY INGREDIENTS TO
BEING MAGNIFIQUE
INSIDE & OUT

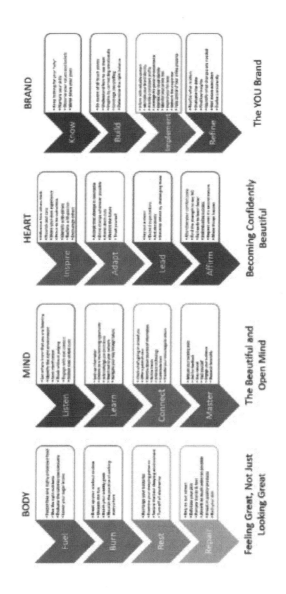

EXERCISE TEMPLATE

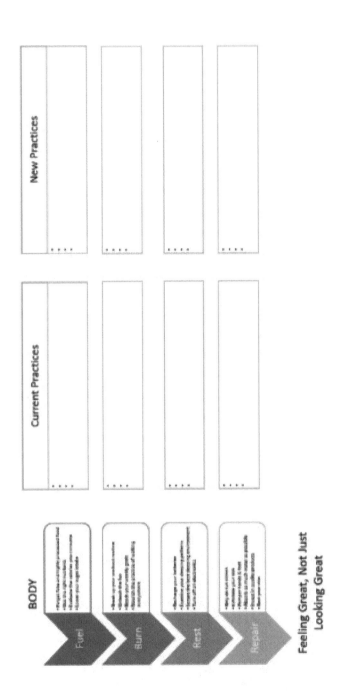

New Practices

Current Practices

BODY

Fuel

Burn

Rest

Repair

Feeling Great, Not Just Looking Great

EXERCISE TEMPLATE

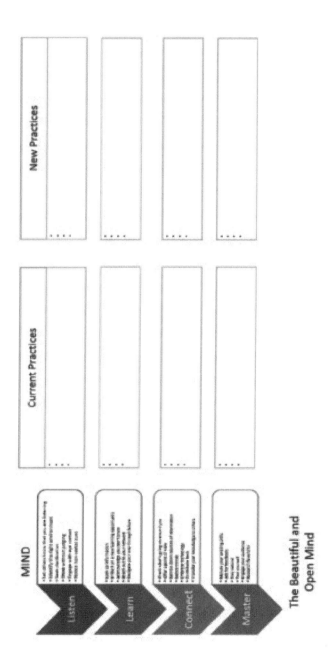

EXERCISE TEMPLATE

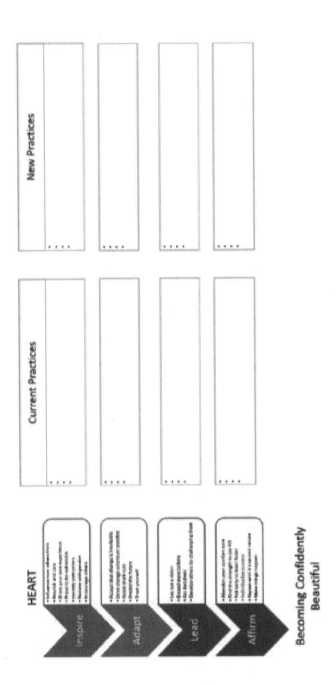

EXERCISE TEMPLATE

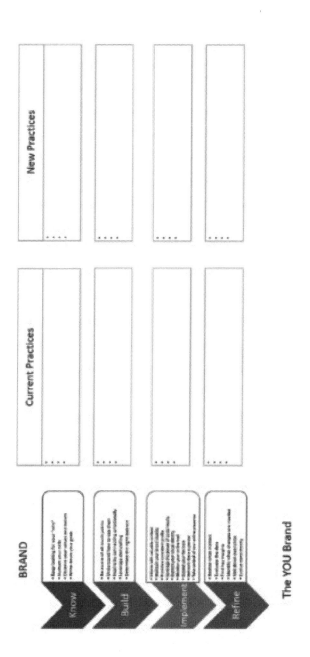

NOTES

Introduction

Heidi D'Agostino, Nancy Etcoff, Susie Orbach and Jennifer Scott, "The Real Truth about Beauty: A Global Report," Findings of the Global Study on Women, Beauty and Well-Being, Commissioned by Dove®, a Unilever Beauty Brand, 2004.

Penn Schoen Berland, "Perceptions of Beauty," 2014. Survey responses collected from September 10-14, 2014.

Chapter 1: Are We Beautiful and We Just Don't Know It?

"Science of Sex Appeal," Discovery Channel, accessed September 28, 2014, http://www.discovery.com/tv-shows/other-shows/videos/other-shows-science-of-sex-appeal-videos.htm.

"America the Beautiful," http://americathebeautifuldoc.com/atb.html.

Tanzina Vega, "Beauty Might Not Be Blind, but the Casting Call Was," *The New York Times,* September 1, 2011.

Bare Escentuals website, http://www.bareescentuals.com/.

Beauty Mark website, http://www.beautymarkmovie.com/.

"Belle Toute Nue," http://www.m6.fr/emission-belle_toute_nue.

Chasing Beauty website, http://www.chasingbeautyfilm.com/Chasing_Beauty.html.

Wikipedia, "Dove Evolution advertisement," http://en.wikipedia.org/wiki/Evolution_(advertisement).

Duncan Macleod, "Dove Evolution in Campaign For Real Beauty," October 21, 2006, The Inspiration Room, http://theinspirationroom.com/daily/2006/dove-evolution/.

Dove® Research, "The Real Truth About Beauty," 2004.

Dove® Research, "The Real Truth About Beauty: Revisited," 2010.

"Dove® Self-Esteem project," http://www.dove.us/Social-Mission/default.aspx and http://www.dove.co.uk/en/Our-Mission/Self-Esteem-Toolkit-and-Resources/default.aspx.

"Dove® Real Beauty Sketches," https://en.wikipedia.org/wiki/Dove_Real_Beauty_Sketches, Dove® official website, http://realbeautysketches.dove.us/.

Tanzina Vega, "Ad about Women's Self-Image Creates a Sensation," *The New York Times,* April 18, 2013, http://www.nytimes.com/2013/04/19/business/media/dove-ad-on-womens-self-image-creates-an-online-sensation.html?.

Emma Gray, "Dove's 'Real Beauty Sketches' Ad Campaign Tells Women 'You're More Beautiful Than You Think'" (video), *The Huffington Post,* accessed April 17, 2013, http://www.huffingtonpost.com/2013/04/15/doves-real-beauty-sketches-ad-campaign-video_n_3088071.html.

Vivian Diller, "Ashley Judd and the Beauty Paradox: A No-Win Situation for Women?," *The Huffington Post,* April 16, 2012, http://www.huffingtonpost.com/vivian-diller.../ashley-judd_b_1425490.html.

David Griner, "H&M Winning Raves for Having a Normal-Looking Woman Model; Its Beachwear Jennie Runk Gets Starring Role," *AdWeek,* May 7, 2013.

"Retouching is 'Excessive' Says Slimline Covergirl Kate Winslet," *Hello!,* January 10, 2003, http://www.hellomagazine.com/film/2003/01/10/katewinslet/.

Brooke Eaton, "Kate Winslet Says You Don't Have to Be a Size 2," *Fox. News,* June 4, 2012, http://magazine.foxnews.com/food-wellness/kate-winslet-says-you-dont-have-be-size-2.

Wikipedia, "Killing Us Softly," http://en.wikipedia.org/wiki/Jean_Kilbourne.

Miss Representation website, http://www.missrepresentation.org/.

"Ashley Judd's Puffy Face Explained," *US Weekly,* March 14, 2012.

"Kate Winslet, Rachel Weisz and Emma Thompson Form 'British Anti-Cosmetic Surgery League'," *HuffPost Celebrity,* accessed October

17, 2011, http://www.huffingtonpost.com/2011/08/17/kate-winslet-rachel-weisz-emma-thompson-form-british-anti-cosmetic-surgery-league_n_929435.html.

"Ashley Judd Slaps Media in the Face for Speculation over Her 'Puffy' Appearance," *The Daily Beast,* Smack-down, April 9, 2012.

"Beyond Stereotypes," Dove Global Study, 2005.

Raj Persaud, Consultant Psychiatrist, Maudsley Hospital.

Chapter 2: The Pearl in All of Us
All quotations from the individuals below are from the following timeframe:

Brittany Dawn Brannon, March/April, 2013.

Connor Boss, March/April, 2013.

Heidi Forrest, April/May, 2013.

Kristen Dalton, March-May, 2013.

Marika Siewert, April/May, 2013.

Maureen Francisco, April/May, 2013.

Melanie Kannokada, July/August, 2013.

Susie Castillo, March-May, 2013.

Kristen Dalton, *Rise Up, Princess: 60 Days to Revealing Your Royal Identity* (Kristen Dalton Wolfe, 2014)

Chapter 3: Recipe for Success
All quotations from the individual below are from the following timeframe:
Lola White, April/May, 2013.

Chapter 4: Feeling Great—Not Just Looking Great

Wikipedia, "Hope Solo," http://en.wikipedia.org/wiki/Hope_Solo.

Nick Eaton, "Hope Solo Tells Her Compelling Story in Upcoming Autobiography, *Seattle PI*, July 24, 2012, http://blog.seattlepi.com/seattles-ports/2012/07/24/hope-solo-tells-her-compelling-story-in-upcoming-auto-biography/.

Piper Weiss, Shine Staff, "Highs and Lows of Olympic Soccer Star Hope Solo," *Yahoo! Shine Canada,* July 27, 2012, https://ca.shine. yahoo.com/blogs/healthy-living/highs-lows-olympic-soccer-star-hope-solo-195600913.html.

Robert Klemko, "Hope Solo: 10 Things You Might Not Know," *USA Today,* accessed July 28, 2012, http://usatoday30.usatoday.com/sports/olympics/london/soccer/story/2012-07-27/10-things-you-might-not-know-about-hope-solo/56555898/1.

Jill Lieber Steeg, "Solo's Success as USA's Goalie Is No Accident," *USA Today,* accessed July 25, 2007, http://usatoday30.usatoday.com/sports/soccer/national/2007-07-24-hope-solo_n.htm.

GerrySpratt,"HopeSoloGracesCoverofESPNtheMagazine'sBodyIssue," *SeattlePI,*October5,2011,http://blog.seattlepi.com/thebigblog/2011/10/05/hope-solo-graces-cover-of-espn-the-magazines-body-issue/.

Carly Schuna, "Can You Eat Too Many Fruits & Vegetables?," accessed January 8, 2014, http://www.livestrong.com/article/261132-can-you-eat-too-many-fruits-vegetables/.

Mayo Clinic staff, "Water: How Much Should You Drink Every Day?" accessed October 10, 2014, http://www.mayoclinic.org/healthy-living/nutrition-and-healthy-eating/in-depth/water/art-20044256.

Gina Shaw, "Water and Your Diet: Staying Slim and Regular With H2O," http://www.webmd.com/diet/features/water-for-weight-loss-diet.

Russell Foster, "Why Do We Sleep?" TEDGlobal 2013, http://www.ted.com/talks/russell_foster_why_do_we_sleep?language=en.

American Psychological Association, *2010 Stress in America Report.*

Cameron Russell, "Looks Aren't Everything. Believe Me, I'm a Model." TEDxMidAtlantic, October 2012, http://www.ted.com/talks/cameron_russell_looks_aren_t_everything_believe_me_i_m_a_model.

Stephen Adele, "Expert Trainer, An Exclusive Interview With Carla Sanchez," accessed September 2014, http://www.isatori.com/44-Expert-Trainer.aspx.

Sandra Aamodt, "Why Dieting Doesn't Usually Work," TEDGlobal 2013, http://www.ted.com/talks/sandra_aamodt_why_dieting_doesn_t_usually_work?language=en.

Mireille Guiliano, *French Women Don't Get Fat: The Secret of Eating for Pleasure* (New York: Vintage, 2007).

Michael Pollan, *In Defense of Food: An Eater's Manifesto* (New York: Penguin, 2009).

Susan M. Kleiner, *Power Eating,* 4th Edition (Champaign, IL: Human Kinetics, 2013).

Susan M. Kleiner, *The Good Mood Diet: Feel Great While You Lose Weight* (New York: Grand Central Life & Style, 2007), Kindle edition.

David L. Katz, *Disease-Proof: The Remarkable Truth About What Makes Us Well* (New York: Hudson Street Press, 2013).

Marion Nestle, *Food Politics: How the Food Industry Influences Nutrition, and Health,* revised and expanded edition (Oakland: University of California Press, 2007).

Marion Nestle, *What to Eat,* New York: North Point Press, 2007.

United States Department of Agriculture, http://www.choosemyplate.gov/.

Lou Schuler, Cassandra Forsythe and Alwyn Cosgrove, *The New Rules of Lifting for Women: Lift Like a Man, Look Like a Goddess* (New York: Avery Trade, 2008).

Cassandra Forsythe, *Women's Health Perfect Body Diet: The Ultimate Weight Loss and Workout Plan to Drop Stubborn Pounds and Get Fit for Life* (Emmaus, PA: Rodale, 2008), Kindle edition.

Cassandra Forsythe-Pribanic, "Are Government Guidelines Making Us Really Fat?" June 2, 2011, http://www.cassandraforsythe.com/web-articles.

Wikipedia, "Julianne Hough," http://en.wikipedia.org/wiki/Julianne_Hough.

"Favorite Recipes and Healthy Living Tips," accessed September 2014, http://juliannehough.com/.

Esther Crain, "Julianne Hough's Secret Workout Weapon," *Women's Health,* February 25, 2014.

Wikipedia, "Padma Lakshmi," http://en.wikipedia.org/wiki/Padma_Lakshmi.

Patty Adams Martinez, "Padma Dishes It Out," *Fitness Magazine,* November 2013.

Sam Dean, "What Top Chef's Padma Lakshmi Eats for Breakfast," *Bon Appetit,* May 28, 2013, http://www.bonappetit.com/people/article/what-top-chef-s-padma-lakshmi-eats-for-breakfast.

Lee Spencer, "Female Drivers Know Value of Gym Time," Fox Sports, updated June 6, 2014, http://www.foxnews.com/sports/2012/06/20/cup-female-drivers-know-value-gym-time/.

Karla Walsh, "Race Car Driver Danica Patrick Talks Home Fitness Favorites and the Cause Close to Her Heart," *Fitness Magazine,* February 15, 2012.

Wikipedia, "Danica Patrick," http://en.wikipedia.org/wiki/Danica_Patrick.

Wikipedia, "Lindsey Vonn," http://en.wikipedia.org/wiki/Lindsey_Vonn.

Patty Adams Martinez, "Olympic Skier Lindsey Vonn's Lower-Body Workout," *Fitness Magazine,* February 2011, http://www.fitnessmagazine.com/workout/real-plans/celebrity/lindsey-vonn-workout/.

Amy Van Deusen, "Lindsey Vonn's Interview," *Women's Health,* accessed September 28, 2014, http://www.womenshealthmag.com/fitness/lindsey-vonn.

Nathaniel Vinton, "Olympic Star Lindsey Vonn Trades Racing Uniform for Bikini in *Sports Illustrated* Swimsuit Issue," *New York Daily News,* updated February 10, 2010, http://www.nydailynews.com/sports/more-sports/olympic-star-lindsey-vonn-trades-racing-uniform-bikini-sports-illustrated-swimsuit-issue-article-1.194769.

Lindsey Vonn website, accessed September 28, 2014, http://www.lindseyvonn.com/en/home/.

Nilofer Merchant, "Got a Meeting? Take a Walk," TED 2013, http://www.ted.com/talks/nilofer_merchant_got_a_meeting_take_a_walk?language=en.

National Sleep Foundation, accessed September 28, 2014, http://sleepfoundation.org/.

American Psychological Association, accessed September 28, 2014, www.apa.org.

Arianna Huffington, "How to Succeed? Get More Sleep," TEDWomen 2010, http://www.ted.com/talks/arianna_huffington_how_to_succeed_get_more_sleep?language=en.

Russell Foster, "Why Do We Sleep?" TEDGlobal 2013, http://www.ted.com/talks/russell_foster_why_do_we_sleep?language=en.

Wikipedia, "Serena Williams," http://en.wikipedia.org/wiki/Serena_Williams.

Deborah Bennett, "Serena Williams Endorses Sleep Sheets, Designed To Beat Insomnia," *Hello Beautiful,* May 3, 2012.

Dorkys Ramos, "Serena Williams Reveals Problems with Insomnia and Relationships," bet.com, updated May 1, 2012, http://www.bet.com/news/fashion-and-beauty/2   012/05/01/serena-williams-reveals-prob-lems-with-insomnia-and-relationships.html.

Lindsay Goldwert, "Tennis Star Serena Williams Endorses Sleep Sheets, Dissolving Strips with Melatonin, to Beat Insomnia, *New York Daily News,* May 3, 2012, http://www.nydailynews.com/life-style/health/tennis-star-serena-williams-endorses-sleep-sheets-dissolving-strips-mel-atonin-beat-insomnia-article-1.1071462.

Jessica Cumberbatch Anderson, "Serena Williams Tackles Insomnia as Co-Owner of 'Sleep Sheets' Sleep Aids," *The Huffington Post,* updated May 10, 2012, http://www.huffingtonpost.com/2012/04/30/serena-wil-liams-tackles-sleep-problems-with-sheets_n_1465015.html.

Serena Williams website, accessed September 28, 2014, http://serenawilliams.com/.

SleepIQ by Sleep Number, accessed September 28, 2014, http://www.sleepnumber.com/sleepiq/.

National Sleep Foundation, "Inside Your Bedroom-Use Your Senses," accessed September 28, 2014, http://sleepfoundation.org/bedroom/.

Wikipedia, "Allyson Felix," http://en.wikipedia.org/wiki/Allyson_Felix.

Allyson Felix, "Olympic Gold & Silver Medalist, Eight-Time World Champion Sprinter, ACUVUE® Celebrity Mentor & paid ACUVUE® Spokesperson," accessed September 28, 2014, http://www.beauty.com/guest-editor-allyson-felix/qxc297591.

Lauren Drago, "Q & A with Pro Sprinter Allyson Felix," *Teen Vogue,* accessed September 28, 2 014, http://www.teenvogue.com/beauty/health-fitness/2011-07/interview-with-allyson-felix/?slide=1.

Allyson Felix website, accessed September 28, 2014, http://www.allysonfelix.com/.

Unilever, "10 Tips for Even More Beautiful Skin," accessed September 28, 2014, http://www.unileverusa.com/brands-in-action/detail/10-Tips-for-even-more-beautiful-skin/301724/.

Wikipedia, "Christie Brinkley," http://en.wikipedia.org/wiki/Christie_Brinkley.

Christie Brinkley website, accessed September 28, 2014, http://christiebrinkley.com/.

Jessica Prince, "Beauty Diaries: Christie Brinkley," *Harper's Bazaar,* March 14, 2014.

"Christie Brinkley Dishes on Her Skincare Secrets," *Fox News Magazine,* April 21, 2014.

Kate Sullivan, "Allure Beauty Diaries: Maria Menounos Never Reapplies Makeup and Re-Uses False Eyelashes," September 12, 2011, http://www.allure.com/beauty-trends/blogs/daily-beauty-reporter/2011/09/the-allure-beauty-diaries-maria-menounos-never-reapplies-makeup-and-re-uses-false-eyelashes.html.

Wikipedia, "Maria Menounos," http://en.wikipedia.org/wiki/Maria_Menounos.

Robin Hilmantel, "Beauty Tricks Maria Menounos Swears By," *Women's Health,* June 25, 2013.

Alex Apatoff and Suzanne D'Amato, "Maria Menounos's Surprising (and Surprisingly Elaborate) Trick to Get Perfect Skin," February 7, 2014, http://stylenews.peoplestylewatch.com/2014/02/07/maria-menounoss-surprising-trick-to-get-radiant-skin/.

Andrea Lavinthal, "Maria Menounos Shares Her Best Beauty Tips," *Cosmopolitan,* March 30, 2009, http://www.cosmopolitan.com/style-beauty/beauty/how-to/a8026/maria-menounos-beauty-tips/.

"Maria Menounos' Favorite Products from Her Book-The Everygirl's Guide to Life," November 12, 2012, Celebrityfavs.com.

Maria Menounos, *The EveryGirl's Guide to Life* (New York: It Books, 2011).

Maggie New, "Why Is Mineral Oil Bad for Your Skin?" updated June 20, 2014, http://www.livestrong.com/article/185370-why-is-mineral-oil-bad-for-your-skin/.

The Skin Cancer Foundation, accessed September 28, 2014, http://www.skincancer.org/.

Google Consumer Multiple Answer Survey, completed October 7, 2014, by 200 women in the U.S. on the Google Consumer Survey network. Answers were displayed in random order.

Chapter 5: The Beautiful and Open Mind

Wikipedia, "Sara Blakely," http://en.wikipedia.org/wiki/Sara_Blakely.

Kathy Caprino, "10 Lessons I Learned from Sara Blakely that You Won't Hear in Business School," May 23, 2012, http://www.forbes.com/sites/kathycaprino/2012/05/23/10-lessons-i-learned-from-sara-blakely-that-you-wont-hear-in-business-school/.

Robert Frank, "Billionaire Sara Blakely Says Secret to Success is Failure," October 16, 2013, http://www.cnbc.com/id/101117470.

"Spanx Founder Sara Blakely Dared to Ask, 'Why Not?'," video, http://www.inc.com/sara-blakely/how-sara-blakley-started-spanx.html.

Brainy Quote, Sara Blakely, accessed September 28, 2014, http://www.brainyquote.com/quotes/authors/s/sara_blakely.html.

Sara Blakely, "The Road to Entrepreneurship Wasn't Easy," accessed September 28, 2014, http://www.spanx.com/-cms-spx_saras_story_20130613_150822.

Wikipedia, "Alfred Binet," http://en.wikipedia.org/wiki/Alfred_Binet.

Ryan Jaslow, "Video Captures 40-Year-Old Woman Hearing for the First Time," March 28, 2014, CBS News, http://www.cbsnews.com/news/40-year-old-joanne-milne-hears-for-first-time/.

"Deaf Woman Joanne Milne Hears for First Time," March 28, 2014, BBC, http://www.bbc.com/news/uk-england-tyne-26779079.

Evelyn Glennie, "How to Truly Listen," TED2003, http://www.ted.com/talks/evelyn_glennie_shows_how_to_listen?language=en.

Julian Treasure, "5 Ways to Listen Better," TEDGlobal 2011, http://www.ted.com/talks/julian_treasure_5_ways_to_listen_better.

Wikipedia, "Michelle Kwan," http://en.wikipedia.org/wiki/Michelle_Kwan.

Michelle Kwan, *Michelle Kwan: Heart of a Champion: An Autobiography* (New York: Scholastic Trade, 1997).

Wikipedia, "Jennie Finch," http://en.wikipedia.org/wiki/Jennie_Finch.

Jennie Finch website, accessed September 28, 2014, https://www.jenniefinch.com/.

Wikipedia, "Kristen Stewart," http://en.wikipedia.org/wiki/Kristen_Stewart.

Kristen Stewart website, accessed September 28, 2014, http://www.kristenstewart.com/.

Amanda Fortini, "Kristen Stewart-ELLE's June Cover Girl on Relationships, Privacy, and Her Critics," *Elle*, May 5, 2010.

"Oprah Winfrey: Entrepreneur, Host and Philanthropist, Simple Reminders," Post 291 of 370, accessed September 28, 2014, http://simplereminders.com/20140304101411.html.

Wikipedia, "Scarlett Johansson," http://en.wikipedia.org/wiki/Scarlett_Johansson.

Brainy Quote, Scarlett Johansson, accessed September 28, 2014, http://www.brainyquote.com/quotes/authors/s/scarlett_johansson.html.

"Scarlett Johansson Fever Strikes Again," *The Independent*, April 13, 2010.

Google Trends, accessed September 28, 2014, https://www.google.com/trends/.

Wikipedia, Kelly Clarkson, http://en.wikipedia.org/wiki/Kelly_Clarkson.

Kelly Clarkson website, accessed September 28, 2014, http://www.kellyclarkson.com/.

Toastmasters International, "10 Tips for Public Speaking," accessed September 28, 2014, http://www.toastmasters.org/mainmenucategories/freeresources/needhelpgivingaspeech/tipstechniques/10tipsforpublicspeaking.aspx.

Wikipedia, "Adele," http://en.wikipedia.org/wiki/Adele.

Brainy Quote, Adele, http://www.brainyquote.com/quotes/authors/a/adele_2.html.

Adele website, accessed September 28, 2014, http://www.adele.tv/.

Robyn Hatcher, *Standing Ovation Presentations*, (Carlsbad, CA: Motivational Press, 2013).

Google Consumer Multiple Answer Survey, completed October 7, 2014, by 200 women in the U.S. on the Google Consumer Survey network. Answers were displayed in random order.

Chapter 6: Becoming Confidently Beautiful

Miguel Helft, "Sheryl Sandberg: The Real Story," *Fortune Magazine,* October 10, 2013, http://fortune.com/2013/10/10/sheryl-sandberg-the-real-story/.

David de Jong, "Sheryl Sandberg Becomes One of Youngest U.S. Billionaires," Bloomberg, January 21, 2014, http://www.bloomberg.com/news/2014-01-21/sheryl-sandberg-becomes-one-of-youngest-u-s-billionaires.html.

Sara Nathan, "From Teenage Aerobics Instructor to Facebook's Billion-Dollar Woman and Is the Next Stop the White House? The Astonishing Rise and Rise of Sheryl Sandberg," Daily Mail, March 1, 2013, http://www.dailymail.co.uk/news/article-2286584/Facebooks-Sheryl-Sandberg-teen-aerobics-instructor-COO--stop-White-House.html.

Wikipedia, "Sheryl Sandberg," http://en.wikipedia.org/wiki/Sheryl_Sandberg.

Sheryl Sandberg, Makers Profile, accessed September 28, 2014, http://www.makers.com/sheryl-sandberg.

"Sheryl Sandberg Addresses the Class of 2012," Harvard Business School, May 24, 2012, http://www.youtube.com/watch?v=2Db0_RafutM.

Sheryl Sandberg, *Lean In: Women, Work, and the Will to Lead* (New York: Knopf, 2013).

Wikipedia, "Alexis Wineman," http://en.wikipedia.org/wiki/Alexis_Wineman.

Wikipedia, "Lizzie Velásquez," http://en.wikipedia.org/wiki/Lizzie_Vel%C3%A1squez.

Rebecca Savastio, "Watch the 'World's Ugliest Woman' Blow Your Mind," January 10, 2014, Guardianlv.com, http://guardianlv.com/2014/01/watch-the-worlds-ugliest-woman-blow-your-mind-video/.

Mishal Husain, "Malala: The Girl Who Was Shot for Going to School," BBC News, October 7, 2013, http://www.bbc.com/news/magazine-24379018.

Wikipedia, "Malala Yousafzai," http://en.wikipedia.org/wiki/Malala_Yousafzai.

Malala Fund, accessed September 28, 2014, http://www.malala.org/.

Malala Yousafzai, *I Am Malala: The Girl Who Stood Up for Education and Was Shot by the Taliban* (New York: Little, Brown and Company, 2013).

Shehryar Taseer, "Malala, The Bravest Girl in the World," *Newsweek,* October 29, 2012.

Robert B. Cialdini, *Influence: The Psychology of Persuasion,* revised edition (New York: Harper Business, 2006).

Dale Carnegie, *How to Win Friends & Influence People* (New York: Pocket Books, 1998).

Experience Project, accessed September 28, 2014, http://www.experienceproject.com/.

Brené Brown, "The Power of Vulnerability," TEDxHouston, June 2010, http://www.ted.com/talks/brene_brown_on_vulnerability?language=en.

John Green, *The Fault in Our Stars* (New York: Dutton Books, 2012).

"This Star Won't Go Out," accessed September 28, 2014, http://tswgo.org/.

Wikipedia, "Lara Logan," http://en.wikipedia.org/wiki/Lara_Logan.

Lara Logan 60 Minutes, 60 Minutes Sports correspondent, co-host Person to Person, Bio, CBS News, Jun 24 2014, http://www.cbsnews.com/team/lara-logan/.

Wikipedia, "Emma Thompson," http://en.wikipedia.org/wiki/Emma_Thompson.

The Helen Bamber Foundation, http://www.helenbamber.org/.

Wikipedia, Kate Middleton, http://en.wikipedia.org/wiki/Catherine,_Duchess_of_Cambridge.

The Duchess of Cambridge, the official website of the British Monarchy, accessed September 28, 2014, http://www.royal.gov.uk.

The Royal Foundation, accessed September 28, 2014, http://www.dukeandduchessofcambridge.org/.

Wikipedia, "Charles Darwin," http://en.wikipedia.org/wiki/Charles_Darwin.

The Good Judgment Project, accessed September 28, 2014, https://www.goodjudgmentproject.com/.

Wikipedia, Melissa Stockwell, http://en.wikipedia.org/wiki/Melissa_Stockwell.

Melissa Stockwell website, accessed September 28, 2014, http://www.melissastockwell.com.

Wikipedia, Lupita Nyong'o, http://en.wikipedia.org/wiki/Lupita_Nyong'o.

"Lupita Nyong'o Delivers Moving 'Black Women in Hollywood' Acceptance Speech," February 28, 2014, http://www.essence.com/2014/02/27/lupita-nyongo-delivers-moving-black-women-hollywood-acceptance-speech/.

"Lupita Nyong'o on Her Magical Journey from Kenya to '12 Years A Slave' and Possible Oscar Glory," *The Daily Beast,* February 22, 2014.

"Lupita Nyong'o Delivers an Incredible Speech on Beauty: 'I Prayed to God for Lighter Skin," March 06, 2014, http://www.news.com.au/entertainment/celebrity-life/lupita-nyongo-delivers-an-incredible-speech-on-beauty-i-prayed-to-god-for-lighter-skin/story-fn907478-1226846866664.

Wikipedia, "Gabrielle Reece," http://en.wikipedia.org/wiki/Gabrielle_Reece.

Gabrielle Reece website, accessed September 28, 2014, http://www.gabbyreece.com/.

Gabrielle Reece, *My Foot Is Too Big for the Glass Slipper: A Guide to the Less Than Perfect Life* (New York: Scribner, 2014).

Sally Jenkins, "Pat Summitt, Tennessee Women's Basketball Coach, Diagnosed with Alzheimer's Disease," *The Washington Post,* August 23, 2011.

Wikipedia, "Pat Summitt," http://en.wikipedia.org/wiki/Pat_Summitt.

Pat Summitt Foundation website, accessed September 28, 2014, http://patsummitt.org/.

Katty Kay and Claire Shipman, *The Confidence Code: The Science and Art of Self-Assurance—What Women Should Know* (New York: Harper Business, 2014).

"*The Confidence Gap* by Katty Kay and Claire Shipman," *The Atlantic,* April 14, 2014.

Wikipedia, "Bethany Hamilton," http://en.wikipedia.org/wiki/Bethany_Hamilton.

Bethany Hamilton website, accessed September 28, 2014, http://bethanyhamilton.com/.

Bethany Hamilton, *Soul Surfer: A True Story of Faith, Family, and Fighting to Get Back on the Board* (New York: MTV Books, 2006).

Wikipedia, "Dara Torres," http://en.wikipedia.org/wiki/Dara_Torres.

Dara Torres website, accessed September 28, 2014, http://daratorres.com/.

Dara Torres, *Age Is Just a Number: Achieve Your Dreams at Any Stage in Your Life* (New York: Three Rivers Press, 2010).

Bobby Bakshi, *The 101% You: Seven Steps to Creating the Life of Your Choice* (Seattle: Self-Publishing, 2010).

Immaculée Ilibagiza, *Left to Tell: Discovering God Amidst the Rwandan Holocaust* (Carlsbad, CA: Hay House, 2007).

Aimee Mullins, "My 12 Pairs of Legs," TED2009, http://www.ted.com/talks/aimee_mullins_prosthetic_aesthetics?language=en.

Aimee Mullins, "Changing My Legs-and My Mindset," TED1998, http://www.ted.com/talks/aimee_mullins_on_running?language=en.

Wikipedia, "Aimee Mullins," http://en.wikipedia.org/wiki/Aimee_Mullins.

Aimee Mullins website, accessed September 28, 2014, http://www.aimeemullins.com/.

Google Consumer Multiple Answer Survey completed October 7, 2014, by 200 women in the U.S. on the Google Consumer Survey network. Answers were displayed in random order.

Chapter 7: Developing the "YOU" Brand

Wikipedia, "Oprah Winfrey," http://en.wikipedia.org/wiki/Oprah_Winfrey.

Mia Mask, "Oprah: The Billionaire Everywoman," NPR, March 4, 2010, http://www.npr.org/templates/story/story.php?storyId=124285128&from=mobile.

"Nike Launches 'Find Your Greatness' Campaign," accessed September 28, 2014, http://news.nike.com/news/nike-launches-find-your-greatness-campaign-celebrating-inspiration-for-the-everyday-athlete.

David Gianatasio, "Nike Looking for Greatness in Ordinary People and Places. Olympic-timed Work, for Once, is Celeb-Free," *AdWeek,* July 26, 2012, http://www.adweek.com/adfreak/nike-looking-greatness-ordinary-people-and-places-142207.

Wikipedia, "Angelina Jolie," http://en.wikipedia.org/wiki/Angelina_Jolie.

Wikipedia, "Jennifer Aniston," http://en.wikipedia.org/wiki/Jennifer_Aniston.

Wikipedia, "Rick Warren," http://en.wikipedia.org/wiki/Rick_Warren.

Rick Warren, *The Purpose Driven Life* (Grand Rapids, MI: Zondervan, 2002).

Wikipedia, "Adam Leipzig," http://en.wikipedia.org/wiki/Adam_Leipzig.

Adam Leipzig, "How to Know Your Life Purpose in 5 Minutes," TEDxMalibu, February 2013, http://tedxtalks.ted.com/video/How-to-Know-Your-Life-Purpose-i.

Wikipedia, "Tina Fey," http://en.wikipedia.org/wiki/Tina_Fey.

Wikipedia, "Jessica Alba," http://en.wikipedia.org/wiki/Jessica_Alba.

Gerald Olivier, "Jessica Alba Biography, IMDb Mini Biography," accessed September 28, 2014, http://www.imdb.com/name/nm0004695/bio.

Wikipedia, "Keira Knightley," http://en.wikipedia.org/wiki/Keira_Knightley.

Keira Knightley Biography, accessed September 28, 2014, http://keiraknightleyfan.com.

Wikipedia, "Ellen DeGeneres," http://en.wikipedia.org/wiki/Ellen_DeGeneres.

Lacey Rose, "The Booming Business of Ellen DeGeneres: From Broke and Banished to Daytime's Top Earner," *The Hollywood Reporter,* August 22, 2012, http://www.hollywoodreporter.com/news/ellen-degeneres-show-oprah-winfrey-jay-leno-364373.

Pierre Thoretton, *L'amour Fou,* performed by Yves Saint-Laurent and Pierre Bergé (2010; France: Les Films du Lemdemain, USA release 2011), DVD.

Wikipedia, "Beyoncé," http://en.wikipedia.org/wiki/Beyonc%C3%A9.

Beyoncé website, accessed September 28, 2014, http://www.beyonce.com/.

Wikipedia, "Michelle Sung Wie," http://en.wikipedia.org/wiki/Michelle_Wie.

Michelle Wie website, accessed September 28, 2014, http://michellewie.com/.

Google Alerts, accessed September 28, 2014, https://www.google.com/alerts.

Wikipedia, "Lila Tretikov," http://en.wikipedia.org/wiki/Lila_Tretikov.

Wikimedia, "Lila Tretikov Profile," accessed September 28, 2014, https://meta.wikimedia.org/wiki/User:LilaTretikov_(WMF).

Wikipedia, "J. K. Rowling," http://en.wikipedia.org/wiki/J._K._
Rowling.

Joanne Rowling website, accessed September 28, 2014, http://www.
jkrowling.com/.

Google Consumer Multiple Answer Survey completed October 7,
2014, by 200 women in the U.S. on the Google Consumer Survey network. Answers were displayed in random order.

Conclusion

Dan Ariely, *The Upside of Irrationality: The Unexpected Benefits of Defying
Logic* (New York: Harper Perennial, 2011).

Wikipedia, "Banteay Srei," http://en.wikipedia.org/wiki/Banteay_Srei.

Wikipedia, "Liv Tyler," http://en.wikipedia.org/wiki/Liv_Tyler.

All quotations from the individual below are from the following
timeframe:

Elizabeth Lindsey, July 2014.

Zakiya Jamal, "Colbie Caillat Wants You to 'Take Your Makeup
Off'," video, *People,* July 11, 2014, http://www.people.com/article/
colbie-caillat-try-video.

Sharon Tanenbaum, "Colbie Caillat's 'Try' Video Makes You
Feel Beautiful—and Might Make You Cry," *US Weekly,* July 15, 2014,
http://www.usmagazine.com/entertainment/news/colbie-caillat-
tearjerker-try-video-sends-powerful-message-2014157.

"You Are Beautiful," accessed September 28, 2014, http://you-are-
beautiful.com/.

Wikipedia, "The Little Prince," http://en.wikipedia.org/wiki/The_
Little_Prince.

Antoine de Saint-Exupéry, *The Little Prince* (New York: Mariner
Books, 2000).

Photographs by iStock (Getty Images)

50968152R00183

Made in the USA
Columbia, SC
14 February 2019